A Woman's Journey Offers
Insight & Guidance for Optimal Health at Any Age

Looking for Health in All the Right Places

Putting Together Life's Puzzle Pieces

ANNIE SCHEPPACH

Looking for Health in All the Right Places

To contact the author, visit
www.AnnieScheppach.com

ISBN-10: 1532740727
ISBN-13: 978-1532740725
LCCN: 2016906390
Createspace Independent Publishing Platform

Printed in the United States of America

Cover Design: Katherine Lambert

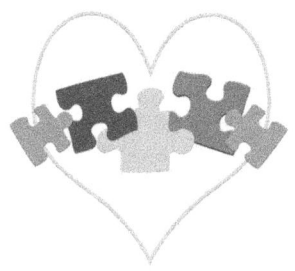

courage (n.) c. 1300, from Old French *corage* (12c., Modern French *courage*) "heart, innermost feelings; temper," from Latin *cor* "heart," from PIE root, which includes Sanscrit, **kerd-* (1) "heart" (see ***heart*** (n.)) which remains a common metaphor for inner strength. In Middle English, used broadly for "what is in one's mind or thoughts," hence "bravery," but also "wrath, pride, confidence, lustiness," or any sort of inclination.

Paying It Forward

Please know the proceeds from this book will be contributed to research and dissemination of information of ways in which "Comprehensive Lifestyle Practices" may ease side effects children experience when undergoing treatment for cancer, and to help reduce recurrence of secondary cancers later in life for children treated with current therapies.

I have so much gratitude for the many advances in treatment of acute lymphoblastic leukemia. Children, like my grandson, Ryan, diagnosed January 1, 2013 at seven years, eleven months old, and treated with chemotherapy, which I choose to view as a liquid gold elixir for him, much love, and prayer for three years and three months, now have an opportunity to do what kids do...

Love, laugh, play, learn, and grow up to their greatest potential.

Praise for

Looking for Health in All the Right Places

I picked up Annie's book fully intending to read a few pages. Instead, she captured my attention immediately from the first few words. And I could not put this amazing book down. Annie glows in real life, and this is reflected in her extraordinary life journey. Her book is practical and walks you through her ongoing discoveries about her own health and what "health" really means. The depths of her spiritual re-awakening will have you searching for yours. I feel her love of life and her intensity and commitment to reach for optimal health. Wherever you are in your life, from the novice who is looking to simply get better to the most seasoned holistic teacher, I highly recommend this book. Read it now if you feel something is missing in your life.

-Dawn Beltz, ND

You are taking your gift for inspiring people to take charge of their lives, their health in a whole new way, to the printed page. Your readers will discover, as I have, that you are a wonderful life teacher, a role model. And when they follow your guidance, I am sure they will find their health improves too.

-Sharon Armstrong, Sharon Armstrong and Associates

Annie Scheppach has been ahead of her time for decades, often thinking "outside the box." Based upon her independent study of prevention of chronic diseases and wellness, she offered a proposal during our tenure at the Social Security Administration (SSA) that had the potential of saving large sums of the Federal trust funds and at the same time for helping thousands of individuals on the SSA disability roles to live healthier lifestyles. We should have given her recommendations greater consideration. But readers of her book have a chance to benefit from her wisdom.

-Richard Eisinger, former Senior Executive Officer,
Social Security Administration

"The intro chapter is incredible! I lost myself in reading about your experience. When I finished, I realized that it was a meditative experience for me. It resonated with me to my core and caused an adrenaline surge I felt while reading the final paragraph. I am dying to read more!

It is an egregious understatement for anyone to say that Annie deserves praise for writing this book. It was a courageous act for her to take ownership of the words God spoke to her that day on the beach. That she documented the divine directive and her ensuing journey of personal healing in these pages is truly a heroic achievement meant to fulfill her calling as an inspiration to, and guide for, others seeking to reclaim their health."

- Anne M. Stewart, MD

The author is a graduate of the Institute for Integrative Nutrition, where she completed a cutting edge curriculum in nutrition and health coaching taught by the world's leading experts in health and wellness. I recommend you read this book and be in touch with Annie to see how she can help you successfully achieve your goals.

- Joshua Rosenthal, MScEd, Founder/Director, Institute for Integrative Nutrition

Dedication

For my family who continues to teach me about love and myself.

My children Kris and Ray, who from a young age learned about change and courage and lives fully lived, no matter what.

My extraordinary grandsons Ryan and Sean, who also early on in their young lives have embraced all that life brings – the challenges and the joys. And for their mom Tracey, who loves her boys more than any grandmother could wish for.

For all my teachers and many friends who have held me when the going got tough and played and laughed with me all these years. Their wisdom, love, patience, and acceptance are reflected in whom I have become and continue to become with my "beyond-the-comfort-zone" life.

In memory of Ron, who offered me the gift of myself, and of Kleo, my four-legged companion of eleven years. She meditated and practiced yoga with me and purred me through the heart breaking and heart opening moments.

And for all the readers of this book. May these words written from my deepest heart after so many years of study and self-study guide you and support you in creating your health…for life.

Contents

Autobiography in Five Short Chapters

1.   I walk down the street.
   There is a hole in the sidewalk
   I fall in.
   I am lost...I am hopeless.
   It isn't my fault.
   It takes forever to get out.

2.   I walk down the same street.
   There is a deep hole in the sidewalk.
   I pretend I don't see it.
   I fall in again.
   I can't believe I'm in the same place.
   But it isn't my fault.
   It still takes a long time to get out.

3.   I walk down the same street.
   There is a deep hole in the sidewalk.
   I see it is there.
   I still fall in...it's a habit.
   My eyes are open.
   I know where I am.
   It is my fault.
   I get out immediately.

4.   I walk down the same street.
   There is a deep hole in the sidewalk.
   I walk around it.

5.   I walk down another street.

-Portia Nelson

The Wakeup Call

Twenty years ago, when someone asked, "How are you?" my answer was, "Fine." Isn't that how nearly everyone answers that question? They say, "fine," or, "I am okay," when inside there is often a struggle simply to get through another day. I figured, rightly or wrongly, no one wanted to hear the details of my story. I was not "fine."

I like to use the 10-point scale to assess how I am feeling, even to this day, because the scale requires me to really tune in and listen to what my body is saying. Back to twenty years ago, I was only a 2 or 3 at the most on the 10-point scale, but as I said, I did not think anyone wanted to hear the details. I woke up each morning, often after restless sleep, gazing at the clock, and thinking that in fourteen hours I could be back in bed! What a way to live! I was exhausted—a single mom with an executive level job that included a daily round trip commute of more than a hundred miles in lots of traffic.

I had been given my new dream job, yet I felt my shoulders were not broad enough to cope with the volume of sensitive issues and political machinations. At the same time, my lovely daughter was facing a serious drug problem, and I was worrying about aging parents. Add to that list my own physical and emotional concerns: Allergies, chronic digestive issues (trouble digesting life, although I did not understand the connection then), chronic muscle aches and pains, a long recovery time from uterine surgery (surgery I believe I might have avoided if I had lived my life then as I have learned these past life-changing years), chronic sleeplessness, chronic low level depression, and frequent colds and flus. Oh, did I say dizziness too? I hid it all well. Get the picture? Can you relate in some ways of your own? Today, my answer to, "How are you?" is, "Fabulous." And I really mean it. I even receive some surprised looks with this reply. How did I get from a 3 to a 9 or 10?

What happened next? When I added how I was feeling to knowing one of those birthdays ending in a zero was fast approaching, I recognized I had to do something, but what? In my case, what else but a late fall vacation? Where? Well, being too busy to give it much thought (wait, wasn't that a part of the problem?) and no time to find anyone to go with me, I chose Club Med in Cancun. Before you get an impression of a party woman, let me tell you that I was always an early to bed, early to rise woman. I simply wanted a warm beach and a few people to talk with when I wanted to talk!

Early the first morning, a hot and humid November morning, I pulled up a lounge chair on the empty expanse of sand. Why? To meditate. It was to be a first for me. I must have heard a sound bite that meditating was good for stress. I didn't know anyone in those days who meditated. This was over twenty years ago, remember. Our culture placed real value on the brain, action, not feelings.

I hadn't read any self-help books. I probably did not know they even existed. So I closed my eyes, squirmed a bit, whined to myself about the heat and humidity, and noticed my thoughts racing, racing. After only a few minutes...I knew only a few minutes had elapsed because I looked at my watch several times in fifteen minutes, I found myself saying aloud, "This isn't getting me anywhere." My goal was to meditate for fifteen minutes. I found myself saying aloud, "This isn't getting me anywhere." And then a moment I have never forgotten came. I can remember the details today. I heard a voice. Yes, a voice. A male voice by my left ear said, *"Clean the sediment from the pipes."* This was the event that came to divide my life...the before and the after.

Please do not decide this is crazy. You have to know that I was extremely conventional and practical in my thinking and living. I was trying so hard to be the best mom, employee, daughter, and friend. I simply placed too much demand for perfection on myself. Familiar? My body, however, was trying to tell me, *enough already, slow down, take care of yourself in a new way.* But I couldn't really see or feel that then. My behavior was to just keep going, keep pushing, acting as though I were "bulletproof," as my daughter later said. That November week, I only knew that the power and initial strangeness of these words playing over and over in my mind were an accompaniment to the worry, the endless deep exhaustion and aches in my body.

I grew up in Maine in the fifties, and Mainers are people of few words! In my childhood world, we didn't talk about health, as I remember. We did talk a bit about telling no "wrong stories." Mom would not even let us use the word "lie." There were a few conversations about kindness, snow, fear of polio, and the Russians attacking, building bomb shelters or hiding under our desks, but we did not talk about God, much less about hearing voices. I never explored religion or spirituality in all the intervening years. Maybe I prided myself like many sixties generation people I knew on believing there was no God, or at least believing that if I could not see "it," "it" probably did not exist. Yet, immediately upon receiving this message, I just knew without a doubt that I had been given a gift, well, actually a warning as well. And the magnitude of this gift I could not explain. I did know there had been no other human being on that beach. I had even abruptly opened my eyes and looked around, thinking I might see someone, yet knowing I would not. Was that my Maine practicality? All of this occurred in a split second. These words echoing and echoing, *"Clean the sediment…"* were not words anyone I knew would say, except perhaps a plumber!

I could have ignored the words, just created a story around them and kept on going. As I reflect back today, I wonder if I would still be alive, much less thriving, as I am, if I had not heeded the "wakeup." I had to change everything that I was feeling. And that was followed with, "Okay, Ann (I was Ann in those days), now what are you going to do?" It was not until much later that I understood that my variety of symptoms over the years were in fact mini wakeup calls, and that this message on a Cancun beach was the strongest one yet. It got my attention. Not for a moment did I consider ignoring those words. Really, there was no question that I had received the gift of possibility, a new life—a healthy, vibrant life. I questioned over and over during that week, and over the years to come, what I was supposed to do next while replaying the words, *"Clean the sediment from the pipes."*

Words that, for years, I shared very selectively. You can guess why! What you are holding is a brief guide filled with what I believe will support you in achieving extraordinary wellness—the guide that I wish I'd had. It includes what I know works because I have done and continue to live what I am offering you. In this book, I share pieces of my story, of healing, of creating a new life, my life after the wakeup. In essence, an "autobiography" of sorts in five chapters. These chapters contain the basics, the pieces of a puzzle to guide you to feeling fabulous and so alive.

For these twenty plus years, I have devoted my life to the intense study of health, of living. Such a change in the mid-stream of life, and so early in the movement of nourishing self-care, raised lots of eyebrows. My kids, for example, did not understand this mom who was no longer the mom they grew up with, and they wondered why this ongoing commitment and passion was my life. Now, these adult children, who are about the same age as I was when I received the wakeup, look at me and sometimes ask my advice. I have gone to schools for certifications, to retreats, taken so many classes on health, and more. My bookcase is filled with hundreds of books including the newer ones written by doctors who increasingly have realized that the conventional medical model generally is not so effective in treating the epidemic of chronic disease. Yes, doctors are daring to speak up. And I, like the doctors, have found my voice over the years.

Now in my seventies, yes, I do feel fabulous. Mostly, I am a 10 on that 10-point scale I mentioned earlier, and gratefully, take no medicines. I live what I have written here. I just had to say that again.

I continue to learn because I love it. It is *never too late or too early to make your health a priority*. Should I repeat that too? It is *never too late or too early to make your health a priority*. Are you ready? Are you open to new ideas that may challenge you? Will you be open to making new choices? To tweaking your current choices? Your choices in each and every moment, right now, can lead to a dramatically healthier, happier outcome for you and possibly for those you love. What I do know from my journey to super health and happiness, and from the paths of so many others, is that we must make health a priority in our busy lives now. Living in a body that feels great is such a reward for giving it loving attention. And, yes, avoiding and perhaps healing chronic diseases is the flip side of the coin. This is an inside job. I invite you to choose to make it fun.

For several years, I have known I had to write this book for you. I understood the book was not so I might become famous. I simply had to write this book to inspire you. My nudge to offer you this story, this how-to book, I can no longer ignore. Can you ignore the nudge that led you to holding this book? May all of you create the life you are meant to live no matter your age, or no matter where you are on the 10-point scale in this moment. This is my gift to you when you are ready—my knowledge of *"if I had known then what I think I know now."*

What is Happening?

"All truth passes through three stages:
First, it is ridiculed;
Second, it is violently opposed;
Third, it is accepted as self-evident."

-Arthur Schopenhauer

B efore we get into the big picture of health and wellness (or is it disease we mostly talk about), ask yourself, "What is happening in my life? How am I really feeling in my body, my mind, my heart, my spirit?" Yes, all of this! Have you ever stopped to ask yourself these revealing questions? We often take our health, our life, for granted. As for happiness, do you take that for granted too? Or do you even ask yourself if you are happy? And isn't it all tied together? Some of us are unaware until.... Yet, we know at the same time, that hard stuff happens to all of us.

Just as I became clear that I had to do something following little nudges, then lots of not so little nudges, and then the big one so long ago...nudges that led to changing my way of life completely, ask yourself what nudges are you ignoring? Are you willing to pause, take some deep breaths, and be so honest with yourself? What is the number on the 10 point scale for you? Make a commitment to yourself to read this book with an open mind, not a, "This is absurd—there is not enough time in my busy life and mind." Also, resist thinking one of the biggest myths: "I could never be this healthy. It is all genetic." You know the way your mind works at the moment. I promise you can fabulous at any age. In the event you missed these words before, you are never too young or too old, nor is it ever too early or too late to make your health and your family's health a priority. By the way, disease begins years before there are any symptoms. My beliefs and your beliefs, instilled by our parents, their parents, our culture, all that we are exposed to from the time we were children, have led us to making millions of choices up to this moment—the vast majority of which are, undoubtedly, serving us well. Yet, many beliefs about health are based upon myths, even lies. Your understanding may shift significantly from this point forward. Remember that people used to believe the world was flat. Let's get going.

8 Myths Most of Us Grew up With*

1. "My mom had it. My dad had something else. I am doomed." I met a former colleague who said exactly that over lunch one day. She was not open to hearing anything that could change her belief. The science of epigenetics proves this FALSE with a capital F. Instead, know that lifestyle trumps genes ninety-five percent of the time. What if I told you that you can control turning your genes off and on with your choices?

2. "Pasteurized milk is good for you and your bones." This is an advertising myth propagated by the processed food industry. Advertising.

3. "Whole wheat breads are a great choice." Advertising.

4. "I will lose weight with artificial sweeteners." Advertising.

5. "Hand sanitizing sprays kill most bacteria." More advertising. This one I have to explain here. While it is true that they kill most of the germs, the ingredients in these products add to the toxic load in the body unless you purchase the "clean" essential oil hand sprays from a health foods market. Soap and water are effective if you wash your hands carefully.

6. "If I just exercise enough, I will lose weight."

7. "I have to accept that it is just a part of getting older to have _____ or to take _____." (You fill in the blanks.) Doctors I used to go to always played the "getting older" card that I intuitively discarded! Doctors or their nurse practitioners look up in amazement (or is it disbelief?) when I reply to, "List all the medications you are taking," with, "None."

8. "Everyone has 'it'—a cold, the flu, headaches." No, it is the immune system, the stressors, which are the key factors here. When our immune systems are strong, we don't get what "everyone has." The "everyone has it" is just a way to be like the ostrich, to keep living the way you are living and not look within to question if there is anything you can be doing differently.

You will discover why I consider these myths as you read this book!

Big Picture - A Little Bad News Before the Good News

There is a chronic disease epidemic in this country. Nearly fifty percent of the adult population has at least one diagnosed chronic disease, seventy percent take one prescription drug, and twenty percent take five or more[1]. The United States spends more on health than any other country, and we are not even ranked in the top twenty for life expectancy, and only fifteenth for happiness[2]. Might there be a correlation between health and happiness? Eighteen cents of every dollar we spend is spent on chronic disease management ($9,255 per person)[3]. What is it costing you? (And not just in dollars.)

Do you know anyone who does not have one chronic condition? Addiction, Alzheimer's, arthritis, allergies, asthma, back pain, cancer, Crohn's or other digestive conditions, depression, diabetes, fibromyalgia, headaches, heart disease and stroke, obesity, oral health concerns, Parkinson's. Unfortunately, the list goes on and on. While our healthcare system is extraordinary when it comes to the practice of acute medicine, it falls exceedingly short when it comes to preventing and healing chronic conditions. Yet, a change is beginning in the thinking about health in this country. While not yet a tidal wave, I predict with a smile that a new wave of thinking is coming. Leading edge doctors, too, are discovering there is another way and are writing about healthy living after discovering that patients typically don't heal if they follow the conventional dogma of the last seventy-five years. In the meantime, there will be those who continue to scream quackery and those who resist a change in our understanding. Large corporations, which make billions on illness, spend millions to fight the truths that are now being written and talked about by people like myself, doctors, and scientists. One voice is being added to another and another. The conversation and the research is shifting as a new paradigm is becoming self-evident that many healthier alternatives are available to us for living this one precious life.

Four Big Picture Truths - The Good News. In My Opinion

1. Every chronic disease is generally preventable and reversible! (Read this again and again.) The message of the medical world and echoed by the media has been one of early diagnosis and managing chronic disease. To know there is a possibility of preventing and reversing a disease is freeing, YES! My preferred emphasis, it almost goes without saying, is to focus on all the work that prevention and lifestyle require, so that we never hear those words, "You have…"

2. Every symptom is your body's wisdom trying to get your attention so you will make some changes in your life. YES, changes. When you ignore a symptom, there will be another and another. Think back—is that true for you? And when you take a pill, you are only hiding or masking the symptoms. Of course, if you are on prescription drugs, don't stop the medication after reading this—that could be dangerous. You always need to work with your doctor to change dosages safely. Just know that many of you are able to stop medicines over time. When you have a headache, what do you do? Most people run to the medicine cabinet for a highly advertised, over-the-counter magic bullet, I mean, pill, right? But is your body's wisdom saying, for example, that you have an aspirin deficiency? What is it saying? Maybe rest, breathe, get some water or healthy food. You probably know what your body is telling you if you pause to listen. Your body's wisdom is teaching you, helping you to become aware through aches and pain or illness.

3. You are responsible—response able. We hear about early detection, even a bit about preventive medicine, but not enough on how to get and stay healthy. Embrace that you, not your doctor or the prescription you are holding, are responsible on a day-to-day, moment-by-moment basis for your health and how you feel in your body and mind. Yes, of course, we all need a doctor on our health team. However, dare to question or run from any health provider who acts like a commander when it comes to chronic disease, or who tells you that you have to "live with it."

    Another reason to run is if the doctor says that foods do not matter, or if he only offers you a five or ten-minute office visit before pulling out the prescription pad. Voice of experience here. A health coaching client in the military once told me that at her military doctor's office was a sign which informed patients to only bring up one symptom each visit! Many years ago, I even had a female doctor ask me if I were trying to "kill myself" when I refused a prescription for hormone replacement medication. I did run, and you may know that hormone therapy was found to lead to the heart disease that the therapy was supposed to help prevent. By the way, even with most, but not all cancers, you have a few weeks to research, get an advocate, a cancer wellness coach, and pull together a team in your corner before you start treatment.

4. Contrary to some ads for prescription meds, there is no magic bullet, no surgery without potential dangerous side effects, and no pill for permanent weight loss. Watch out for the sound bites or headlines of any "just released" study that tell you to do just one simple thing or to eat one thing to be healthy. It would also

be wise to question who paid for a study to determine if there is funding bias.

So, What Else Before the Guidance?

"The function of protecting and developing health must rank even above that of restoring it when it is impaired."

-Hippocrates

Before you read this section, please reread the Hippocrates quote. Are you making your health a daily priority, or everything else? Okay, I just had to point it out!

Are you wondering why I have lumped these chronic diseases together? UMMM. Several years ago, I became aware from all the literature I was studying that these diseases are conditions of inflammation. When you read a book about Alzheimer's, a cause behind the cause is inflammation, a book on asthma talks about inflammation, cancer, too, and silent inflammation, and the list goes on—the chronic disease and inflammation link. Where does inflammation come from? Of course, when you get a simple cut, there is inflammation. Inflammation is meant to be temporary. The total stress on the body and the mind builds up and leads to inflammation. Lifestyle. Most chronic disease is from stressors. And where does stress come from? I believe you know the answer—from the foods we eat and more. Yes, foods, not enough sleep, our thoughts and reactions, and too much sitting. These are all things we can change. Another stress factor is the environment. Though we don't hold as much ability to change the environment by ourselves, we must commit to changing what we can. Consider that the total toxic load on your body is the major contributor to the inflammation and sickness in your body.

The burden on our bodies from all the stressors combined is what may tip one into disease. Each of us has a different tolerance point to the cumulative stressors. Really, it is the tipping point. Thus, we have to make more of an effort with the things we can change. The what-to-do to get healthy, to stay healthy, or become even healthier are very much the same no matter the disease. I really hope you take this in. What you can do is outlined in the chapters that follow. With countless books that suggest what to do for a healthier brain, to lose weight, or to help almost any condition, the basics are pretty much the same, no matter what symptoms you are experiencing or the diagnosis. Does that surprise you? Obviously, there is no question that frightening diagnoses like cancer require more attention on your part and your physician's, more quickly and thoughtfully. Just be aware as treatment is outlined that your doctor, in all likelihood, had almost no training in healthy organic foods, mega dose vitamin therapy, or other integrative approaches that may be just what you need to support you in regaining your health. Your doctor may not know about nontoxic ways, or the pros and cons of nontoxic ways, to mitigate some of the side effects of chemotherapy, for example, when chemo has been agreed upon by the patient and the team of doctors as an essential part of treatment.

Start reducing the stressors on your body and mind. Now. What you do today to nourish your body, mind, and spirit creates your future. Remember that your choices determine which genes are fired and which are not. Please reread that last line several times until you don't feel any lingering resistance. AND now, ask yourself, "WHY DO I WANT TO BE HEALTHY? WHAT AM I WILLING TO DO?" What number on the 10-point scale do you intend to be? Remember that it took you years to get where you are. While the health you were born with will return gradually, you will feel changes quickly enough that you will be motivated to continue your new choices for living this one life. Let me remind you—you are never too young or too old. Let's take this a bit further to pre-birth!

Okay, this might be shocking to you. If you are planning to start a family, consider waiting a few months and follow all the steps in this book, or better yet, for the specifically what to do, pick up *The Better Baby Book* to give the new soul you are bringing into this life an opportunity for greater health. Why? Isn't it logical to question if parents who are not extremely healthy can bring in healthy offspring? I can take this further. In the spring, you fertilize the soil, plant the seeds, and water the garden for the vegetables for your table in a few months. Why would you not prepare your "soil" when you are planning a child, the greatest gift of all? *The Better Baby Book,* written by a fertility doctor and her nutrition expert husband, is based in part on epigenetics to affect the environment and expression of the parental genes, and offers information about detoxification, healthy eating, and stress reduction for a healthier baby. If you need a little more reason, consider that studies have shown that the umbilical cords of newborns contain more than two hundred environmental toxins[4].

The next few chapters will show you how to put the pieces of the puzzle together. It is confusing and overwhelming when you see all the books and the headlines saying, "Just do this," whatever "this" is. Who should you believe? Believe yourself first. Also, instead of thinking of this as work or impossible or totally unrealistic, choose to make it an exciting adventure of possibilities. Your choices may be lifesaving for you and your family. Even if you're already in great health, there is always a little more to learn about how to be your own best health insurance. Are you excited about the possibilities?

You will find guidance on getting moving, nourishing foods, cleaning out the cabinets, sleeping, creating healthy thoughts and beliefs, and opening your heart—all of these together represent your answers. Yes, the secret to being oh, so alive.

When I was in a tiny village in Turkey a few years ago, a long-lived couple relaxing in the late afternoon on their porch was asked how old they were. Without hesitation, the softly smiling wife gently replied through the translator, "We've been alive since birth." Are you inspired to begin to take the steps you need to take to become alive your whole life, like this couple was? I even wonder if it is possible to be really alive without the gift of health.

CHAPTER 1

Get Moving, Playfully

"Clear your mind of can't."

-Samuel Johnson

"Whether you think you can or you can't, you're right."

-Henry Ford

Move playfully? When I was little, I heard, "Can't you sit still?" Or, "Don't run." Even, "Stop making faces." "Be careful, dear, you might hurt yourself." "Don't go near the edge." Do you think I ever moved or exercised without cautionary words playing like tapes? My moving was limited to climbing trees when Mom was not looking, and riding a bike in a route carefully circumscribed by her. Besides, I was a girl of the fifties, remember. Girls did not play sports. I think it was considered un-lady-like. And Title IX preventing sex discrimination in sports in schools did not come into existence until 1972, which seems so many lifetimes ago today. Yet, I do remember a ping pong tournament in high school. Since my dad patiently taught me to play ping pong in our basement, I mustered up the courage to participate. I won! My female gym teacher blurted out, "Anna (I was Anna then!), I can't believe you can do anything!" Years later, I was at a management retreat with mostly men and there was a ping pong table. Would you believe I wondered if I should let the men win? For me, it went back to high school and to the cultural stereotypes of allowing men to feel good. I decided it was a new day, and I shone. Do you have a story buried deep inside that may, at some level, be keeping you from moving and moving playfully? Don't dare revert to the "I am too old" story.

While today moving may mean never stopping, such as mindlessly running errands, let's just talk about moving and exercising in the conventional context. Everyone knows to exercise, that exercise is good for you, right? Do you exercise? I began exercising when I was twenty-eight because that was when I initially heard, or maybe was able to hear, about heart research and running for cardiovascular benefits. No one I knew was running the pavements or working out in those days. Today, a great deal of research, including brain research, is discovering the benefits of getting moving, but forty-five years ago (yes, that long ago), I simply got out my Keds and headed outdoors. After a case of shin splints, I acquired running shoes and began to run around the track. I loved being outside. I began running in the neighborhood after the track became boring. I remember a moment, years after I began running, early one morning just before dawn, when I thought, "Oh, this is what the six-million-dollar man or the bionic woman must have felt." For just a breath or two, I had become weightless, suspended in space, so in the moment, feeling invincible as though I could go forever. Then, thinking, thinking came back and the feeling was gone. (It took many years for me to learn the value of being in the moment, and that is another chapter!) I kept running anywhere from two to five miles several times a week. It felt good while easing stress too. Ten years later, I added weight training. I loved both and I loved how energized I felt after a run, a visit to the gym, after a hike in Shenandoah National Park, or after tennis with friends or my young son. Today, I often go out for the P.A.C.E. Run, an interval run where I run fast, well, sort of fast, for thirty seconds, walk for ninety seconds, and repeat eight times, usually!

Moving is healing on so many levels. Just find what you love and go do it. Playfully. Connect with nature whenever you can. When the weather permits, walk barefoot on the grass to benefit from Earth's energies. Run or walk without earbuds so you can hear the birds calling each other or even hear the wind. Smile when you are running or walking. Some people with their hardened facial expressions look as though they are generating more stress as they exercise to reduce stress! One more idea for your running or strength training—look into the high intensity interval training I just mentioned. It only takes twenty minutes! This is a newer practice I've added to my health…for life.

Call a friend. I have a friend who walks with several neighbors at 6:30am each morning, rain or shine, hot or cold. Creating a community supports our intention to get moving, as does a set schedule. Maybe dance, swim, garden, strength train, do aerobics, play basketball, bike, bowl, hula hoop, play ping pong, find a local rec center, or bounce on a trampoline. Purchase a quality trampoline, turn up the music, and set a timer for ten to twenty minutes. Bouncing is so great for the lymphatic system and your mood. You can also try shaking for a few minutes. Shaking helps slow movers to move in the morning and relieves stress any time. Remember this after a stressful meeting. Picture the African gazelle after escaping a lion. The gazelle naturally shakes for a few minutes or so to eliminate stress from its cells. Talk about body wisdom.

Whatever you do, please do not sit hours a day. Are you one of those people who spends half your waking hours sitting? Studies are revealing that sitting for lengthy periods increases your chance of developing diabetes, heart disease, or dying early…even if you exercise. For very sedentary people, the incidence of cancer increases, perhaps dementia too, according to another report[5]. Several years ago, I bought a stand up desk, but I don't just stand there like a statue. I watch my posture, the position of my head and shoulders, and I move around every few minutes. With moving outdoors and in, I generally get at least the recommended 10,000 daily steps, which I used to track with my Fitbit. Sometimes my Fitbit displayed I was an overachiever. Honestly, I have given the overachieving habit up, mostly. Have you? And now my latest discovery: Would you believe I wore my Fitbit for a year, morning and night, also in order to track my sleep, actually enjoying seeing the results? Along came another wakeup one morning! I stared at my orange electronic Fitbit and realized I might be adding unnecessary EMF exposure. For years, I have limited my exposure where I can, based upon my research. How did I not think of this earlier? It was not a beat myself up moment, just an appreciation for the insight. It was so easy to put the Fitbit in the drawer for now. Remember, my intent is to limit the toxic burden on my body where I can.

If you sit a lot or are someone who loves to collapse on the couch, especially at the end of your work day, please reconsider. I often think of my mom who sat or napped on the couch most of the day because she did not sleep well after she retired. Maybe not moving around enough contributed to her not sleeping well. Why did she choose not to move? My dad slouched in his chair beside her, sitting all day, developing aches and pains from not moving. Here is a new diagnosis for the medical world—chronic sitter. I watched them become weaker and weaker, less engaged too early, from this daughter's point of view. I could not change them, nor can I change anyone. What I can do is share what I have learned, and how I've chosen to "age" differently. I am not anti-aging! Yes, we establish so many habits from our families. If your family moved playfully or did not, what do you choose? Finally, no matter what your age, even if you must be in a chair, there are exercise programs for you. Just start any exercise program gradually and notice how you begin to feel so much better.

Are you feeling like you can do this? Or is the way you're feeling holding you back from playfully moving? Or maybe you have had a commitment to exercise for years and still are not feeling as happy and healthy as you would like. Or are you thinking, as I used to, that if you just exercise more, you will feel better?! The BUT. There is a "but." Exercise, I discovered, was not the sole answer to keeping me healthy. That was another myth I no longer needed to subscribe to. You read how I was a 2 or 3 on the 10-point scale in spite of my commitment to exercising at least an hour or more daily. This was a part of the wakeup. There had to be other things I could do to be healthy, or must do to be healthy and alive like the Turkish couple. There had to be more to reducing the stressors on my body and mind.

Have I got the next piece of the puzzle for you! Energy, health, and less inflammation inside and out come from healthy foods. If you are thinking that you already eat in a healthy way, you may be in for a surprise. Are you experiencing an, "Oh no, another thing I have to do," feeling? Are your eyes glazing over in anticipation of the, "Do this and don't do that," or, are you experiencing a sense of relief that the answers to so many of your health concerns are being revealed? We are, after all, putting the puzzle pieces together. While moving is absolutely essential, remember there is no magic bullet. Are you hearing that becoming healthy is about nourishing your body in a number of ways? Nourishing, another word that was not in my vocabulary so long ago, is not limited to exercising. By the way, experience the sound of nourish when you say it aloud. Maybe say, "I choose to nourish my body." Contrast nourish with, "I diet and diet." Different feeling, eh? After Cancun, my next steps to health turned toward how to nourish myself with foods to *"clean the sediment from the pipes."*

CHAPTER 2

First Things First—The Foods That Nourish

"Let food be your medicine and medicine be your food."

-Hippocrates

"The doctor of the future will give no medicine but will interest his patients in the care of the human frame, in diet and in the cause and prevention of disease."

-Thomas Edison

When I made the commitment to myself on that Cancun beach to do whatever it would take to feel better, I could never have imagined the unfolding story you are reading now. Simply, really not so simply, my life became devoted to breaking out of the box of a lifetime of habits and beliefs. Doing this was challenging, healing, and awakening—and continues to this day. Being different made people uncomfortable, especially family and friends who had known me for years. I vacillated between low keying what I was doing and proselytizing—neither of which I recommend today. If I am asked, of course, that is another story!

Where was I to turn after that moment in Mexico? I did not question my commitment to do whatever I needed to do to recover my birthright, my gift of health. My newly discovered intuition directed me to the nearby, recently opened health foods market. Maybe you have heard the often quoted statement, "When the student is ready, the teacher appears." It is true for me, although I wonder if there were many "teachers" whom I did not recognize along the way because I was not paying attention or because I was not ready for what they had to offer me. Today, I am open to people bearing "gifts."

On my very first visit to the healthy foods market after my return from Cancun, a trim fifty-something man walked up to me in the organic vegetables section and announced, "I feel better than I have felt in my life." What would you think if a stranger walked up to you and uttered those words? I never saw him again after he shared his message and gave me the name of his doctor. I really believe now that he was there to gift me with a portion of the next step of the puzzle. My first thought, at the time, was that I was too rushed for small talk. Rushing, rushing. I mentioned this rushing habit earlier—rushing about even planning my trip to Cancun. And where had that rushing gotten me over the years? Following that thought was, "Well, I have never received a pick up line like that." Do you remember the stories about grocery stores being great places to meet singles? There was a grocery store known as the Singles Social Safeway in the Georgetown area of Washington, D.C. So you can see why my thinking went that direction.

It turns out the stranger was a client of a medical doctor who practiced integrative/alternative medicine (a term unfamiliar to me then) near my work place. (Notice I did not use the word patient. Patient is not a term I use because it seems to effectively remove me from the equation, from the concept of partnership.) Remember that I was commuting fifty miles each way then. I would never have gone to this physician if she were not near my office or "geographically desirable," as they say. In her office, not only did I begin to learn how to choose foods very differently, I took the initial baby steps toward regaining my health and my energy. The next steps I chose were to read and read, as I still do. Books and articles on healthy eating had been invisible to me before then. I was not ready.

Before we go further, let's pause (which is a wonderful reminder as a continual practice), and walk down memory lane to when you were a child. What was your favorite food? What is your memory around the kitchen table? For me, I loved walking into our warm, smoky kitchen after trudging home from school with the Maine nor'easter and snow gusting. The smoke meant Mom had lovingly fried chocolate doughnuts with Crisco in the heavy iron skillet! Then, she coated them with granulated sugar after they cooled. Kid heaven. One led to as many more as I could safely sneak from the crock at the top of the basement steps. I have to add this little, not so little, aside—just about a month before she died in her early nineties, she took my hand, and as I was noticing how thin the skin on her hand was, feeling her trembling, my mom mumbled, "I knew you were taking those doughnuts." There had been no preface. The remark seemed to come from nowhere. I was again a child, caught, and I still smile at the memories!

Memories of the dinner table, however, do not leave me feeling soft and fuzzy. Mostly, the atmosphere was tense. The unsaid, the body language was harder than what was said. My dad sat at the head of the table, my mom to his left, and my grandmother, who lived with us during the winter months, was beside her. I sat silently on the other side of the table, and I have to admit, I don't recall where my younger sister sat! Could that be the subject of a book! In any event, my grandmother had false teeth, not uncommon in those days, and they rattled when she chewed! It would be funny to recall if my dad had not been silently fuming, and my mother literally caught in the middle, trying to keep peace. After "supper," in our world, before television came to Maine and before machines that washed dishes, Dad made sure my grandmother, who wanted to help, could not. He felt she did not get the dishes clean enough! Or was he just needing to exert control?

Would you believe I had totally forgotten those memories, or buried them, until about fifteen years ago while I was living in Los Angeles? Because it was a time of inner turmoil, I decided to experiment with group counseling. One afternoon, the wise counselor brought up the subject of memories of the dinner tables of our youths. One woman spoke of the laughter and conversation around politics. Then, a brave woman spoke about the stress and silence around her table. I was shocked when old memories became like a movie and tears poured. I could never have imagined or believed, even if someone told me, the effects of stored memories and the pain or trauma we are holding inside. I always tried to be like Pollyanna, the blindly optimistic person. And more "work" helped me to "get" that the lifetime façade had been my unconscious need to please probably everyone.

I tell these stories because while the fun memories are great to recall with a gentle smile, the harder memories are important to uncover, acknowledge, and ask how they are affecting you today in what you eat, how much you eat, and how you react within your own family or with others. Were my memories perhaps still playing a role not only in my addiction to sugar but in how I avoided conflict and tried too hard to do everything perfectly? As you uncover the stories, both those you perceive as positive and the negative ones that may be affecting you today, remember not to judge yourself. This is a self-discovery walk, a self-care walk toward the what, the how, and the when to nourish yourself with your foods.

The What to Eat

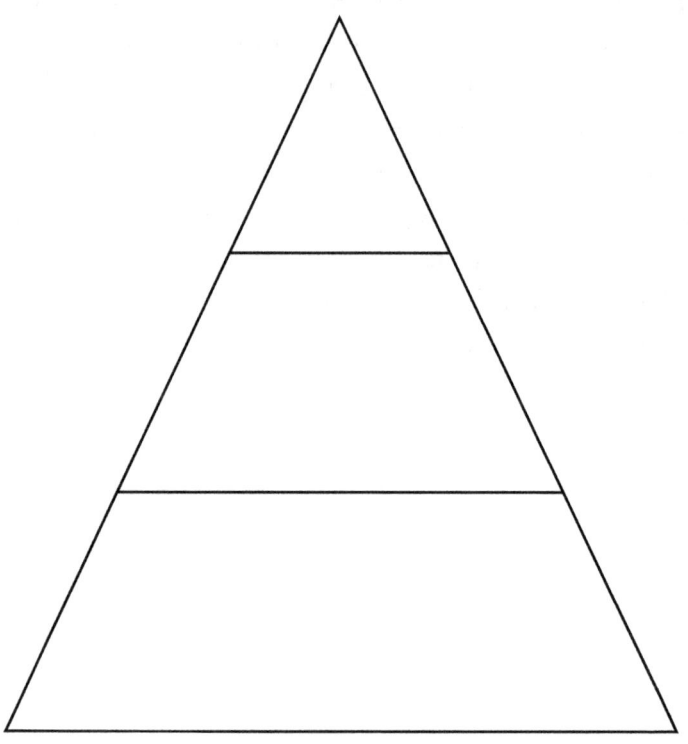

If you like visuals, consider thinking of a pyramid and fill in your own here. The pyramid is a good way to visualize proportions of vegetables, proteins, oils, and nuts.

Foundation of Your Pyramid

Veggies and fruits. Everyone knows this, right? The big question is, "Do you follow this guidance?" Choose mostly veggies because fruits are higher in sugar. Lots of veggies, all the colors of the rainbow. Choose organics for many reasons, including that they have more taste and they are more nutrient dense. In addition, organics contain no genetically modified organisms (GMOs). In light of the science from all over the world that is revealing why GMOs are dangerous, I chose years ago to avoid GMOs. Some countries have banned them, while in our country, concerned individuals are working so hard to have GMOs labeled, at a minimum. Corporations are working just as hard to ensure they are not labeled! If you need another reason for choosing the organic label, know that bug killing pesticides on the non-organics raise hormones in your body, kill the healthy gut bacteria that you need to thrive, and overall, contribute to the toxic burden on your body.

Yes, organics cost more (I can read your mind here), but what is the price tag on your health and the health of your family? Have you heard the expression, "Pay the farmer now or the doctor later?" Talking about farmers, you might choose to save by going to the local farmers' market in season. Another benefit of the market is that the produce will be fresher. It will be a fun adventure too! Another way to save is by opting out of your daily non-organic coffee at the coffee shop, the junk snacks in the machine down the hall in the office, or the packaged goods you normally buy at the grocery store. Thus, you save in one place to purchase the higher quality organics. Right here, I will offer the mantra that the leading edge Institute for

Integrative Nutrition coined, "Get out the chemicalized, artificial, highly refined junk food." HOWEVER, if you cannot afford organic, do not let this stop you from eating veggies and fruits! Just soak your produce in room temperature water mixed with a little white vinegar for ten minutes. Use three-parts water to one-part vinegar and rinse well with non-tap water.

Maybe these stories will inspire you. In Italy, there is a campaign in middle schools to promote healthy eating based on organics. Meals prepared using organic produce were served in over 1200 cafeterias in 2014, with 1.2 million school meals served daily that contained some organics. There is more focus on organics throughout Asia. Uzbekistan has announced a ban on GMOs in baby food. In France, teaching children about healthy food in the classroom and the school restaurant begins when children start school at age three. Only water is served and there is a national ban on vending machines in all schools. The French Ministry of National Education requires that children sit at the table in the school dining rooms for at least thirty minutes to allow them to eat slowly. (The French do not use the term "cafeteria" for the schools' dining places.) What if we did that at home! Yes, a worldwide change is happening.

Level Two of Your Pyramid

Proteins. I choose grass-fed red meat from cattle, lamb, or bison. Pricier, again yes, and healthier, a big yes. Why step up? The cattle from the huge CAFO (Concentrated Animal Feeding Operation) lots are raised on grains, injected with hormones to make them grow faster, and then administered antibiotics because they are sick. Why are they sick? Their living conditions are horrible, and the grains are not what their bodies are made to eat. Whew! Is that a reminder for us that when we eat foods our bodies are not designed to eat of what we may be setting ourselves up for? Those hormones injected into the cattle only for the economic benefit of the grower get into our systems, creating too much estrogen. You are probably familiar with antibiotic resistance in humans. The drugs given the cattle end up in us. A vicious cycle, some might say, and an example of everything being connected to everything.

Wait, there are more benefits to choosing meat from animals which are grass-fed their entire lives and are not grain finished. Even a little grain used to fatten the animal changes their whole fatty profile, and thereby, the health benefits for us. These 100% grass-fed animals, compared to the CAFO animals, are good sources of a healthier ratio of omega-3 fatty acids to omega-6, a higher source of B vitamins, thiamin and riboflavin, higher in calcium, magnesium, and potassium. Omega-3 lowers our body's inflammation markers, the stressors, and isn't that what we have been focusing on, directly and indirectly, in this book? *The British Journal of Nutrition* reported a study where volunteers ate either grass-fed or conventionally raised beef for four weeks. Those who ate moderate amounts of grass-fed for four weeks raised their levels of omega-3, while those who ate the conventionally raised meat saw an increase in omega-6.

Why care? Our bodies make all the essential fatty acids but these two, which we must get from our diets. Unfortunately, in our country, with the high consumption of processed foods, we get way too much of the inflammatory omega-6. They must be in balance, so it is not as though one is bad. Most experts agree that the ratio should be about 1:1. The reality is that the omega-6 may be 20:1 or 50:1 for so many of us.

Enjoy pastured chicken and wild caught fish—not farm raised for reasons similar to those for choosing grass-fed meats. Generally, I only purchase a small amount of wild caught salmon because of its price, but it is the cleanest fish. Most salmon is farm raised, and again, there is the issue of what some are calling Frankenfish—GMO fish that is not labeled. Cold water fish such as wild salmon, sardines, herring, and mackerel are good sources of omega-3 too.

Eggs from pastured chickens are another great source of protein, AND the yolks are rich in beneficial omega-3. Labels here are confusing. "Free-range" only means not caged and doesn't clarify what the chickens are fed. Natural means almost nothing. And eggs are good for you.

If you are a vegetarian, or if you enjoy beans, purchase a wide variety of organic beans from the bins in your favorite health foods market for a great source of protein and a very inexpensive meal. You might soak them before cooking to make them more easily digestible. The caveat is that beans are higher in carbohydrates. Other sources of protein include hemp and chia seeds, nuts, and some of the super foods, including moringa. Bee pollen is 40% protein and one of nature's most complete foods. A little is an excellent addition to your morning smoothie. As for soy, another vegetarian protein source, try organic tempeh, miso, or natto as sources of fermented foods for the gut. When ads for soy mention that Asians eat lots of soy, the truth is that they are generally eating fermented soy as a condiment. Because soy affects estrogen metabolism and because almost all soy in this country is GMO, avoid excessive amounts, including highly processed soy milk with an organic label. Limit the highly processed almond and rice milks in cartons, even if they are organic. I will not forget the highly regarded Dr. Andy Weil saying, "Why would you eat or drink anything in a Tetra Pak?" He was referring to "dead food" with a long shelf life. In addition, soy is on the highly allergenic list for some people. To choose or not to choose soy may require more reading on your part.

Level Three of Your Pyramid.

Healthy fats are at the top of the pyramid. Fats got such a bad rap for so many years! And look what has happened to so many of us. Did you know that fats are essential for your brain health? Many people I know still have the low fat mindset and are fueling themselves on sugar and white stuff—you know, the white breads, pastas, and cookies as opposed to healthy fats.

Draw a vertical line at the top of your pyramid. On one side are your oils—coconut oil and olive oil are my favorites. Purchase them in glass, not plastic, first cold pressed and organic so the oils are clean, not rancid before you pick them up off the grocery store shelf. Coconut oil, neither an omega-3 or omega-6, is very beneficial for your heart, metabolism, immune system, skin, and thyroid. I use it when I sauté any foods because it can withstand a higher heat than olive oil. Don't buy the cheap oils heated to high temperatures like sunflower, safflower, and canola oils. These are full of omega 6, which we were just talking about.

The other side of the top of your pyramid are seeds and nuts. Just be careful not to select those roasted in bad fats, at high temperatures, or salted nuts. I remember devouring the salted peanuts in the blue can for years! You know the syndrome of not being able to eat just one handful. Instead, choose a handful of organic, unsalted raw seeds and nuts for a healthy snack. Choose sunflower seeds, sesame seeds, pumpkin seeds, almonds and English walnuts, which are high in omega-3. Chia seeds and freshly ground flax seeds are perfect additions to your smoothies. You will find these in the bins at the healthy markets too. Avocados are an extremely healthy, high fat snack which help to reduce cravings for sugars, as do nuts, seeds, or even a teaspoon of coconut oil.

I Hear You

Where is the dairy? Where are the breads and whole grains on the government's historical pyramid, now known as My Plate? Know that industry plays a powerful role in determining what is recommended for the plate, which is why I created my own pyramid ten years ago after all these years of study and practice.

Even the dairy people are not claiming dairy leads to healthy bones any longer. Remember those moustache ads? The twelve-year Harvard Nurses' Health Study based upon more than 77,000 women revealed that nurses who drank the most milk and consumed the most calcium from dairy foods had more bone fractures than those who rarely drank milk. And for years we were told to drink our milk! If you ingest too much calcium, it is excreted from the bones into the arteries and leads to heart issues[6]. What a delicate balance our bodies must maintain. Did you know that cow dairy is actually very hard for many people to digest? Grocery store yogurt promoted for healthy probiotics contains way too much added sugar. Read the labels, but in general, there are healthier ways to get your probiotics, which we will get to. If you love cheese and know your body is not lactose intolerant and that you are not sensitive to the proteins in dairy, you might taste goat or sheep milks or cheeses. They contain less lactose and smaller fat globules. See how your body reacts. And you might want to consider unpasteurized dairy if you are going to eat dairy. Just read up at realmilk.com.

As for all bread, pasta, pizza, and cereals, know that your body processes these highly refined foods like sugar, so you get the health damaging insulin spikes. What about the message of healthy whole grains we have been fed? There seems to be little question that the proteins, including the gluten protein in wheat, rye, and barley, are difficult for many of us to digest. They are inflammatory—that word one more time. And if you are one of the millions of Americans who suffer from depression, know the brain and gut are linked. Think about it! Corn, while not a gluten, is also an allergen concern for many, thus inflammatory, and is generally found in most stores only as a GMO.

Is the digestibility question because these grains have been so hybridized or genetically modified since the time of our early ancestors? Or is it that the grains our ancestors enjoyed were fermented? Wheat and corn are in just about all processed foods. Is the problem that we eat so much of them? Or is a part of the problem that our small intestine is not like the cow's, which is designed for grasses. Another contributing factor may be that our overall diets over recent years have led to such unhealthy guts that we cannot process grains effectively. Why do I ask these questions? Because we often never pause long enough to question how our food choices are such habits and to notice the impact of these foods on our energy, our health. In my view, the answer to the questions is, "All of the above!" We try to point to the one cause, the magic bullet, often to simplify our lives, when in fact, the cause being multifactorial is more accurate.

Questions have even been raised about another grain we consider healthy, rice, which has been found to contain arsenic residue. It says a lot that the FDA has pointed out that parents consider options other than rice cereal for their child's first solid food for that reason.

If you are going to consume rice, however, *Consumer Reports* has published that basmati rice from California is the lowest in arsenic and rice from Texas the highest; yet, how hard would it be to find the source? Arsenic in brown rice is higher than white, and we have thought white, because it is more highly processed, is not as nutritious as the brown, and thus, chose the brown. Who knew about the arsenic! While I avoid rice cakes and rice milk because they fall into the highly processed category that raises insulin, here is another reason to avoid rice. Opt for the technically "not grains" such as quinoa, buckwheat, and amaranth, which have the additional benefit of being free of gluten and containing less arsenic. Millet, while being gluten-free, suppresses the thyroid. Just try to consume all grains moderately in the form closest to the way nature created them. Recently, I saw an ad for dog food asking if you were still feeding your dog wheat and corn. How interesting that the pet food industry is on to the gluten thing. Have you also noticed that overweight people have overweight pets? Food messages are changing. Are you willing to change?

Let's go a few steps further. Are you an average American who consumes 152 pounds of sugar annually? If there are two products to say a resounding, "NO," to, they are sugar and high fructose corn syrup. But you know that, right? And you still struggle! There is a reason. Sugar is more addictive than crack cocaine, which gives you an idea of how challenging it is to free yourself of the habit. And sugar is in nearly everything that is prepared—even many of the cooked vegetables in the healthy foods market! Why? I can only guess the chef is playing to the taste buds of most of us. I did ask a chef once in a national healthy foods chain why canola oil is used so extensively in their prepared foods. Do you want to guess why? He came up with a variety of reasons which I did not buy. I was not giving up, and finally, he acknowledged, "Price point." Need I say more?

Oh, and then there are the artificial sweeteners like aspartame, Splenda, and Truvia. Don't buy any of them. Do not be taken in by "sugar-free." Don't even buy the ones that say "like sugar" or say they are made from the stevia leaf. You might be taken in by the word stevia in the ad. Stevia, the complete herb, is a wonderful substitute for sugar and these artificial products, but you need the whole leaf for the benefits. All of the processed foods with artificial sweeteners are filled with other chemicals. Did you know that your amazing body wisdom protects itself from these chemicals by creating more fat cells? Moreover, they stimulate your appetite. Haven't you seen very overweight people with several boxes of these highly promoted artificial sweeteners or other "no sugar" drinks in their grocery carts? I assume they just don't know, and like so many of us, are victims of advertising. Also avoid agave because of the processing and its high impact on insulin resistance. Occasionally, choose a little raw local honey, which has antimicrobial and anti-inflammatory benefits.

I am the first to admit, I still struggle with sugar—crunchy chocolate chip gluten-free cookies. Don't believe, however, that gluten-free is synonymous with healthy. There are still the issues of being highly processed and containing sugar! And if you are still leaning toward processed cookies and other processed foods, at a minimum, be aware of the disguises for "sugar" found in products you would never expect such as ketchup and tomato sauce. Fructose, lactose, sucrose, maltose, glucose, dextrose and many other words you can find on SugarScience.org. Just know that sugar affects every body system, organ, tissue, and cell. Sugar contributes to every chronic disease by affecting the immune system. Lots of information exists in print on the "truth about sugar" if you Google these words. Sugar is inflammatory, and inflammation is the hidden cause behind the cause of disease that we are addressing. Consuming a hundred grams of sugar, what you find in a one-liter bottle of soda, causes your white blood cells to be 40% less effective in taking oxygen from the cells, and causes the cells to become more acidic for up to five hours. Yes, an integrative doctor told me this twenty years ago. He said that the immune system is compromised for hours after consuming sugar. And if I have something sugary for breakfast, a sweet at lunch and dinner, I have created an all-day attack on my immune system. I recognize that in spite of being armed with this information how hard it is to say no completely! Just be gentle on yourself and persistent. Greens and healthy fats can stop a craving or overindulgence. Keep a handful of your favorite nuts and seeds nearby—raw organic walnuts, pumpkin seeds, or cashews and Brazil nuts, and combine with an organic date for sweetness. Remember the teaspoon of coconut oil to help stop the craving.

Are you ready for help with the grocery lists? Watch the sodas and the waters with artificial sweeteners or high fructose corn syrup. These are disease in a plastic container or can! I like reading that the sales of full sugar soft drinks are going down as we become more knowledgeable. What I don't like seeing is sales of the drinks with zero calories going up. Develop the habit of reading all of the ingredients in products you are ready to put in your cart. Better yet, avoid the aisles with the boxes and cans. Watch for MSG, carrageenan, dextrose, maltose, actually any chemicals and colorings, and knowingly return them to the shelf. If I were a betting woman, I would bet that the number of packaged goods you purchase will decline sharply when you start to read the ingredients, and when you start to feel so much better eating healthier unprocessed food, perhaps within as little time as two weeks or less. You may find that even though you are spending more for organics and grass-fed meat, your checkout prices may be just about the same because you have banished the processed foods that cost more than you think and stimulate your appetite.

Before moving on, I should mention alcohol too. Women, please, drink no more than one drink per day. That's twelve ounces of beer and the gluten it contains, five ounces of wine, or no more than 1½ ounces of liquor. Consume more than that and the incidence of stroke goes up, especially for people over fifty. Men can have a bit more, but why, really, have any? There are other ways to relax and be social. Besides, what is healthy about beer and hard liquor? If I were to have a drink, I would choose organic red wine if it were available, and if I am totally forthright, maybe one to two margaritas a year if I visit a Mexican restaurant. I am learning not to beat myself up for the once in a great while choices that are not so healthy.

The Ready or Not Experiment

You have just read the basics about foods. Any surprises? Are you seeing the possibilities? Are you able to see this information not as taking what you think you love away, but as a guide to enable you to choose carefully based upon what you are learning and feeling? Yes, begin to be aware, to notice how you are feeling every time after you eat. Keep a record for a couple of weeks. It won't be long before you feel what boosts your energy, or what foods make you sleepy or make you want to eat shortly after your meal. It might also be good to get a food allergy/sensitivity test to help guide you in your new choices. Soon, you may be saving time and money with fewer trips to the doctor.

Here is an experiment offered at the first health seminar I attended long ago. A Georgetown University doctor told the story of how he recommended to a depressed fifteen-year-old client, following a lengthy getting-to-know-you kind of office visit with her and her parents, to stop eating gluten, dairy, corn, sugar, and soy for one month. When she quickly responded, "I can't possibly do that," they negotiated a two-week experiment. Actually, I think that was his plan all along. At the end of only one week, the mom called the doctor and exclaimed, "We have our daughter back!" They were so grateful they had not listened to two previous therapists who wanted to write prescriptions for antidepressants. My clients with any chronic disease or just an overall malaise began to feel better just as quickly when they were willing to commit to themselves. Note the key words, "willing to commit." Are you willing to try for two weeks what is known as the elimination diet the young client followed? I think you will be astounded how foods affect your mood and energy? You can read up on the elimination diet and reintroduction of foods online when you are ready.

Rev Up Your Cells. More Ideas for You.

- Buy sprouts or grow your own. Sprouts have up to a hundred times more enzymes than your raw veggies and fruits.

- Find the unpasteurized fermented foods in the refrigerated section of your grocery store, or ferment your own cabbage, carrots, or daikon radishes. They help support healthy gut bacteria. I will say again that intestinal health is critical to your health for avoiding and healing chronic inflammation. Leading scientists are talking about the super genome: Your genome, your epigenome, and the newest studies are talking about your microbiome—the 100 trillion gut microbes comprising up to perhaps 200 types of bacteria. In fact, 90% of the cells in your body are microbes and bacteria. We need these micro bacteria to digest our food, resist disease, or heal from chronic disease. Hippocrates said 2000 years ago, "Disease begins in the gut." Wisdom of the ancients. AND to keep your microbiome healthy, not only do you require healthy living foods, you need to get moving, sleep well, think good thoughts, meditate, and love all that you are reading here.… the pieces of the puzzle. Are you seeing how the pieces affect the whole today? And beyond! The latest research is suggesting that the microbiome may affect the future of our children and grandchildren and beyond by impacting our genes[7].

- Make bone broth from leftover chicken or meat. Bone broth is one of the healthiest foods and especially beneficial for people who are ill or whose digestives systems are not yet working optimally. You can find recipes online, and the broth is so easy to make that even I make it. The broth is good for your bones because it is rich in calcium, magnesium, and other nutrients. So maybe you skipped over when I said, "Even I make it." While I love to eat in the way I have described, I am not someone who loves to cook. I steam my organic veggies, bake my fish, or lightly sauté my meats in coconut oil and usually add a salad. My way takes about ten to fifteen minutes. I point this out to show that my way is not time consuming if you are imagining being healthy will require a lot of time. On the other hand, if you are like one of my Italian friends who wakes up each morning with visions of cookbooks dancing in her head, you may enjoy finding healthy recipes online or in the books listed at the end of this book. But I can't give you my friend's number!

- Juicing your veggies helps you to eat more veggies and absorb more nutrients. A green juice a day! Here is one recipe for the best juice I have ever made. I can't not share it. And juicing only takes a few minutes. Combine:

  3 celery stalks

  1 Granny Smith apple

  1 cucumber

  fresh ginger

  1 small ripe avocado or banana,

  1 teaspoon organic raw nut butter

  4 kale stalks

  1 date, pitted (optional)

  1 teaspoon or less of moringa. Moringa, a four-thousand-year-old plant, has a strong taste until you are used to it. While it is expensive, it is so healthy and anti-inflammatory with lots of vitamin C, protein, potassium, and more calcium than milk.

Your juicer will create this yummy drink in less than a minute. It might be the best breakfast or lunch ever. It certainly beats orange juice and a bagel, which raise your insulin level and leave you needing an energy boost in a couple of hours. I make less than half the recipe because after the juice is blended, it loses its nutrient value fairly quickly so I don't want to store it. This is why you can save your money and avoid the green juices in plastic bottles in the store. Sip your green drink and don't worry about your mustache. Take a selfie and put on your Facebook page to inspire others!

- Enjoy a <u>little</u> bit of dark 80-85% organic chocolate for dessert. Its tryptophan triggers serotonin release, the feel good hormone.

From the What to the How and When

A little list here may simplify things:

- Drink a glass of water first thing in the morning with a little Braggs raw unfiltered apple cider vinegar or half an organic lemon. This way, you start the day hydrating your body. You might repeat the apple cider vinegar splash to boost your energy for a workout or for even gargling if you feel a sore throat coming on! Speaking of water, be sure to drink half your body weight each day—non-tap water, if possible.

- Choose a luncheon size plate for obvious reasons. No seconds. On your plate will be only a very, very small amount of protein—about the size of your palm, and not piled high either! See, I know how you might be thinking. To be a bit more precise, if you weigh less than 140 pounds, you should have only two to three ounces of protein. Most of us actually get too much protein, and too much stresses the kidneys. Half to two-thirds of the food on your plate should be colorful, tasty veggies.

- Set out your placemats and a candle for one meal. Please turn off the TV.

- Take a few breaths and express gratitude to the earth, the sun, our farmers, everyone involved in bringing the food to your table before you start to enjoy your healthy choices. Thank the food for nourishing you and helping you to be healthy. Please, sit up straight. Oh, you heard that when you were a child! And now, again! Not only does your posture help your digestion, it is empowering to sit tall.

- Put down your fork or spoon as you are chewing. Didn't your mom tell you that repeatedly or did she say to close your mouth when you chew? Slow down and notice your feelings and sensations when you do. This practice offers a lot of benefits, including supporting your digestion. Did you know digestion starts in your mouth and that saliva contains enzymes that chemically break down food? Actually, even thinking about food causes you to start the digestive process. The transformation of a substance into liquid that nourishes you is such a miracle!

- Enjoy your food, taste it, take in the aromas. Whether you are solo or in a crowd, enjoy, gazing outward or looking inward as you nourish your body. Charles Dickens came to this country in 1867 and remarked about Americans bolting down their food and seemingly only eating to fuel their bodies instead of bringing joy to the experience. In my experience, this is still the way for so many. I find myself occasionally hurrying through a meal. My dad used to say when he was alone after my mom died, "I am eating to get it over with!" In retrospect, I have vague memories of the "doing to get it over with" as a part of the way of life in my childhood home. How can I not have been affected unconsciously by this message until I became aware? Today, we may be hurrying to cross all of "it" off the to-do list. Same thing, eh? Another moment for you to remember your stories here? From this moment on, you get to create memories of wonderful conversations and laughter around your table for your families and friends.

- Stop eating before you are full. Or, this may surprise you, when you burp, yes, that's your body's wisdom saying you've had enough.

- Forget the all-day grazing recommendation, unless you have hypoglycemia. Why? Continuous eating is work for your digestive system. Instead, enjoy three meals as our ancestors did. A teacher of mine favors two meals a day. You will have to decide about that one for your body. Try to finish eating three hours before bedtime. The body has a lot of detoxing work to do you while you are sleeping. Digestion is not one of the chores it should have during that time.

- Notice, there is no mention here of what I consider to be a misguided focus on dieting, calories, or weighing portions. I cannot imagine how unappetizing it would be to count calories. When you adopt the way of life described here, the weight will come off. Focus on how you are feeling and intend to feel. Do I need to say more?

My Thoughts Regarding Supplements

I don't believe there is one simple answer regarding supplements. If your digestive system is not working well, you may not absorb your foods or vitamins well. Possibly, vitamins can cause more harm than good if you purchase cheap vitamins that may contain a lot of toxins. Do some research online and get the best your health food store offers. Don't take a supplement simply because you have read it is good for you or because your friends told you about it. Instead, work with someone who is an expert on supplements and on you! I get an annual overall vitamin and mineral level test from SpectraCell Labs so that I know what my body needs. Having said this, essential supplements, in my view, for most of us are:

- Vitamin D3, perhaps the most important supplement, in liquid form. Inadequate vitamin D levels may put you at greater risk for almost all chronic diseases including dementia, diabetes, muscular sclerosis, and breast cancer. Before you start supplementing, get the vitamin D test called 25(OH)D or 25-hydroxyvitamin D. Also, while getting tested, be sure to ask for the C-reactive protein test which will let you know about levels of inflammation in your body. Most of us are deficient in vitamin D. While sunlight between the hours of 10am-3pm, not blocked by sunscreen, is by far the optimal way to get your vitamin D, it is impossible for most of us to do this all year. Get tested at least yearly. This is one of those tests where you don't want to be in the average range, but in the optimal range between fifty and seventy ng/ml. Cancer patients' levels should be higher. As an aside, clients who come to me taking prescription vitamin D often do not see their vitamin D levels improve.

- Vitamin K2, calcium, and magnesium should be checked too when supplementing with vitamin D. Too much calcium, for example, can result in calcium being leached from your bones and into your arteries, leading to heart issues! Supplementation, again, is not so simple.

- Fish oils. This is a harder one to decide unless you test your levels of omega-6 and 3. Refer back to the discussion of omegas. If your omegas are balanced, continue what you are doing without supplementation. If the ratios are out of balance, stop eating all the processed foods, and retest. Only then, if the test reveals a continued imbalance, find the highest quality fish oil. The jury has not come to agreement yet on fish oils, and I can't help but wonder who is paying for which studies. Enjoy the smaller wild caught fish which contain fewer heavy metals. Remember the canned sardines I mentioned earlier? Enjoy them too. Enough omega-9 is easy to obtain from your olive oil. Algae is another source for your omegas. By the way, knowledge is your power. There is a reason for these long heard expressions.

- Vitamin B and C. You can almost never get too much vitamin C!

- Coenzyme Q10, or Coquinol. We make less of this when we get older. If you are taking a statin, CoQ10 is essential because the drug depletes your body further of the CoQ10. More importantly, do your own research on the side effects of statins and the whole cholesterol question. Cholesterol is a building block for your hormones. Sugar is the enemy when it comes to your cholesterol numbers. As you modify your lifestyle, the ratios of what used to be called "good and bad" fats will improve. I recently heard Dr. Mark Hyman saying that seventy studies from nineteen countries found no correlation between saturated fats and heart disease!

- Pre/probiotics. Prebiotics are food for probiotics, and the more prebiotics we eat, the more efficiently live bacteria can work, and the healthier your gut will be. Enjoy raw chicory, raw Jerusalem artichoke, raw dandelion greens, raw garlic, onion and leeks, and raw asparagus and banana. The caveat is if you have SIBO (small intestine bacterial overgrowth), you should check with a specialist. Always start slowly with any pre or probiotics for your body to accommodate the new foods. Sources of probiotics include yogurt, cheeses, and kefir, preferably unpasteurized. The caveat here is if you have a dairy sensitivity. My preference again are the fermented foods you can buy or make. You can also purchase prebiotic and probiotic supplements. How about this? "Bad" bugs contribute to weight gain.

Summary

There is so much information about best "diets." Reread these pages. Try the elimination experiment. I can only provide the information that I know without a doubt will help you move toward better health. You decide whether to jump in or to ease in gradually. Through my private clients, I've discovered that the most motivated people are often motivated by fear. Those who aren't ready often decide they can live with their symptoms rather than "clean the sediment..." Then there are those who have jumped in with a commitment to themselves and transformed their lives in my six-month program. What category do you place yourself in? Please love yourself enough to choose to nourish yourself now with healthy foods... and more.

Ready to Clean out the Cabinets as You Clean up Your Diet?

"The journey of a thousand miles begins with the first step."
-Lao Tzu

Remind yourself that if you do this, if you choose to clean out your cabinets as a gift to yourself, not because I am telling you to, your experience will be substantially different. Besides, you don't have to wait for spring cleaning or for everything to be checked off the to-do list. Do it now, or create a time and put it on your calendar. Decide to devote at least an hour in the kitchen. I promise you that making a commitment to health will be so much easier without processed temptations taking up space on your shelves.

My son once asked me to work with an obese colleague of his without charging. Generally, I subscribe to the advice that you don't give your services away because the client will not value them. Maybe because my son asked, maybe because he was acknowledging my expertise and caring, or maybe because I understood how sick his colleague was, I agreed. She and I spoke over the phone maybe three to four times for an hour or so. She had reasons with each phone call for not being able to follow up on any of my recommendations that she seemed to have agreed with during each phone time, including this cabinet one. While she acknowledged being sick and worried after so many emergency room visits, I understood she was not ready to change. During the last call, she offered that she did not want to deprive her kids of "junk food" by cleaning out the cabinets. I thought that task might be relatively easy for her to do. I tell you about her, not to judge, but to say that change is hard until you can give a resounding, "I have to do something. I am sick and tired of feeling like this."

Now I, myself, did not do this cabinet clean out all at once because I did not have the puzzle pieces that I have now! Depending on your finances, depending upon how you are feeling, you may speed it up or slow it down, do a thorough cleaning or take baby steps. Just be aware of your self-talk with each choice. These steps are pretty easy and not very time consuming. One hour and you are done. By performing the clean out, you are reinforcing your commitment to you. If you keep some of the processed items, which I hesitate to label as foods, in the cabinets, you will be drawn to them in a vulnerable moment. All the while during you clearing, remind yourself that you have a choice in each moment: Raise the toxic burden, the stress on your body, the inflammation, or take steps to reduce it.

- Open all the cabinets and begin to toss the boxes, packages, plastics, and most of the cans, except the canned sardines or anchovies that are so good for you. You might want to glance at the ingredients as you let go. So processed, so many chemicals. Get the kids involved in reading the ingredients—talk about a teachable moment. Toss oils processed at high heat such as the safflower, corn, sunflower, or any oils in plastic bottles. Please recycle so that as you look out for you, you help the earth too. The oils were probably rancid when you put them in your grocery cart due to the light they were exposed to, the heat, and the plastic! You already know to replace them with olive oil and coconut oil. Maybe enjoy a little pumpkin or walnut oil as special treats, but these are a bit pricey.

- Sugar and artificial sweeteners definitely have to go. Just ask yourself: Will this item nourish me? My family? Look at the salt. Be sure your salt is a high quality one like Celtic sea salt or Himalayan salt. The salt in the blue box you have probably seen from the time you were a child is highly processed.

- Toss the Teflon pans and replace them with glass or ceramic. In other words, use pots and pans that are not toxic. And while you are at it, begin to replace your plastic storage containers with glass. Toxic products leech into you. I also suggest you toss the microwave. Did you know that a plugged in, not turned on microwave is still emitting radiation? You might want to buy an inexpensive Gauss meter that allows you to check if you need proof. The studies on microwaves are often kept buried or deemed not media worthy, unfortunately. As if I needed more information beyond the beeping meter, there are enough questions about what the nuking does to the nutrients in food that made it easy for me to ditch. Science confirms cooking with the microwave causes more inflammation, and what is this book about? Reducing inflammation and stressors.

- When you are peeking under the sink, look at all the cleaning supplies, read the ingredients, and replace them with healthier green products for dishwashing and cleaning. You can even make healthy cleaning products easily. Similarly, check the products you use for washing your clothes. Say "no" to air fresheners, especially the ones you plug into the electrical outlets, and antibacterial soaps or hand sprays in your purse. Substitute high chemical hand cleaners with high quality essential oil hand cleaners that are 99.9% effective against common germs. Say "no" to those products that make your clothes fluffy and smell "good," but also just happen to be toxic to the air you breathe and to your skin, which absorbs everything.

- Consider purchasing a reverse osmosis water filter that filters out chlorine, fluoride, and more toxins. Oh, another myth is that fluoride is good for your teeth. The facts are that we would be better off without it, and fluoride does not reduce cavities. Some countries have banned fluoridation of the water supply, and in this country, a number of communities have passed legislation banning it, while others have tried unsuccessfully so far. So many studies reveal the dangers of fluoride. Fluoride lowers thyroid function, may contribute to bone fractures and dementia, sleep impairment by impairing melatonin production; the list of concerns is extensive.

- Are you are still motivated? Take on a bathroom project. Purchase a shower filter that removes chlorine. Replace your vinyl shower curtain with a fabric one because the steam from the hot shower causes a cascade of chemicals to seep into the air from the vinyl curtain. Now, take time to check the bathroom cabinets. In Europe, more than 1,300 chemicals are banned from use in personal care products. In the U.S., only eleven have been banned, as reported by mercola.com. The deodorants with aluminum, nail polishes and polish remover (I finally said, "No," to nail polish), toothpastes with warnings of not to swallow, everything that you put on your hair, your skin, and lips—all may have to go in order to reduce the toxic burden on your body. The talcum powder you may have been using is being linked to ovarian cancer, and there has been at least one successful lawsuit. Hint: Put coconut oil in the bathroom because it is great for the skin, the lips, and even as a deodorant. Imagine all the money you will be saving by using coconut oil instead of pricey creams on your arms and legs. You can use the savings toward new grocery choices. There are so many ways to be creative and healthier.

- Have you read about indoor air quality? According to the EPA, indoor air contains up to five times or more contaminants than outdoor air, occasionally up to 100 times more[8]. Open your windows for even a few minutes daily unless you live in an area of high air pollution. Consider an air purifier. Check your candles. Many of us love candles. The BUT is quality. The best are the unscented 100% beeswax because they help to clean the air. Your inexpensive candles are adding to your body's toxic burden. Your air can feel so refreshing with a diffuser of essential oils. You might also pick up some Boston ivy or English ivy, a spider plant, or aloe, for example, to improve the air. Just check the list of recommended plants, but ensure they are safe for your pet.

CHAPTER 3

Sleep

Now I lay me down to sleep...

D o you remember when you were small, a prayer or other family ritual when someone who loved you tucked you in? Maybe they even smothered you with hugs and kisses and that was the ritual? What a beautiful revelation for me when my nine-ty-three-year-old dad told me, out of the blue a few years ago, that he continued to say those words, *now I lay me down to sleep...,* his entire life before he went to sleep. He also had a few held back tears in his eyes as he named the family members when it came to, *bless...* I was stunned because he had never revealed his feelings and never spoke of prayer. Was it a way to connect with his mom who died when he was a young boy, and with my mom who had passed shortly before, his two daughters, grandchildren, and great-grandchildren? Was this a way for him to be at peace when he went to sleep? I will never know for sure. What I do know about my dad is that he always slept well. I recently reached out to my cousin, whose mom was my dad's sister. She told me her mom always said this prayer too. How heart opening to discover these family traditions so many years into my life! Does my sharing bring up memories, even questions for you? I wonder if I would have even been moved by these stories and connections when I was a young woman. Or is now the time to talk with your family members… oh, I am taking a leap here!

How well do you sleep? Insomnia, according to the National Institutes of Health, affects 50-70 million of us and has been linked to chronic diseases including heart disease and stroke, diabetes, obesity, cancer, and high blood pressure. The American Academy of Sleep Medicine has reported that being deprived of sleep has the same effect on the immune system as physical stress. Do you make sleeping about eight hours a night a priority? Here is a check list that may help support quality sleep.

During the Day

- Get some natural daylight. It helps to set your body's clock. Try getting out for a walk early in the morning and again at noon. To get your body moving, go outside anytime that is convenient. Remember, though, that 10am-3pm is the optimal time for the body to absorb and process vitamin D from the sun. Then there is the question of sunglasses. Light enters the body through the eyes. Your cells require nutrients from live foods and oxygen from the air you breathe, but it is sunlight that fires up your cells. Besides regulating the body clock, sunlight triggers hormones, energy for the cells. For the light to work its magic, keep your sunglasses off for a few minutes. This may seem paradoxical, no glasses, but yes, glasses for glare and protection. The simple win-win is to take them off for a bit to get the benefits and then put them back on for protection. Another tip: Charcoal grey lenses are the best glare blockers!

- Exercise, yes, but not in the evening if you have trouble falling asleep or staying asleep.

Your Bedroom, A Sanctuary

- Love your bedroom and your mattress. Over the years, I have added organic bedding. Remove any clutter in your sleeping space so that when you walk into your room, you already feel serene and ready for sleep. Actually, it is best to not have clutter in your home period. Doesn't clutter stress you?

- Sleep in a very dark room. Even a little light can affect your internal clock. I have new black out shades and I sometimes use a mask. Even a little light says, "Wake up." The optimal temperature for your bedroom is 60-68°F. If you have to get up during the night, avoid turning on a light. If you need light, purchase a little red or orange bulb that you can turn on so that you do not disrupt your sleep with the blue light spectrum.

- If you have an electric clock, move it, along with all other electronic devices, several feet away from you. So many people sleep with their cell phones by their heads. You may want to look more deeply into electromagnetic (EMF) pollution—when you do, you perhaps will choose to not keep your phone in your pocket or in your bra, as some women do, or by your head when you sleep. You may also choose to text more than talk on the phone and you won't put your iPad on your lap. The World Health Organization has reported that cell phones are possibly carcinogenic[9]. I am remembering to unplug my Wi-Fi when I go to bed. A great deal of research is going on regarding our exposure. For many, many years, there were those who claimed cigarette smoking was safe, and there are now those saying EMFs are safe. Maybe these small changes reduce the toxic burden on the body, maybe they don't. I am going with the research that suggests caution. At a minimum, see if these adjustments in your room result in better sleep if you are not sleeping as well as you would like.

- If you currently use an alarm, set the ring for a gentle awakening. You may not require an alarm when you sleep well because you will wake up naturally rested.

- I bet you have heard this before–no TV in the bedroom. And do not bring work into the bedroom either. It is important to preserve your bedroom as a space for relaxing only. Better yet, no work and no computer for a couple of hours before bed. The blue light emitted from the screen affects your circadian rhythm.

Getting Ready for Bed

- Try to go to sleep by 10pm or 11pm at the latest because your adrenals have a lot of recharging to do from 11pm-1am. At the same time, your gallbladder has to eliminate toxins. Plan to keep the same schedule on the weekends too. This becomes one of the easy good habits once you say, "Yes!"

- Avoid fluids for a couple of hours before bed. Experiment with a high protein snack a few hours before bed if you enjoyed an early dinner. Have a piece of fruit to help the tryptophan cross the blood brain barrier. No sugars or grains, but you know that!

- See if a hot shower or sauna helps.

- Say, "No," to sleeping pills. Instead, try herbs or tea like chamomile, valerian, and lavender.

- Write in your journal, or remind yourself of five experiences from your day for which you are grateful. OR, to help open your heart as you drift off into deep healing sleep, I suggest you write your answers to these questions from the teachings of Anges Arrien. Pausing to discover the answer to these questions will take you deeper than perhaps only a perfunctory thanks for your day.

  > What surprised me today?
  > What touched my heart today?
  > What inspired me today?

- Finally, consider being tested at a sleep disorder clinic if your sleep is not restful after all of the above.

Waking Up

- Smile. Take a few deep, slow breaths. Smile again in the mirror. Walk slowly.

- Consider a new practice of waking up a half hour early each weekday to meditate, walk, or journal. One teacher taught me this mantra: WPM—wake up, pee, meditate. Could that work for you? Notice how quickly you answer the question, then ask it again.

- Decide where your attention goes today. It takes commitment and practice to focus on the most important things first.

- One my favorite ways to start the day is derived from the wisdom of Thich Nhat Hanh:

  > "Waking up this morning, I smile.
  >
  > Twenty-four brand new hours are before me.
  >
  > I vow to live fully in each moment and to look at all beings with eyes of compassion."
  >
  > (My advice: Remember to have eyes of compassion for yourself too.)

- It's okay to wake up laughing! Laughter is the best medicine, and a "medicine" most of us don't get enough of. I used to say to my kids, "Is there a thirty-minute funny show on TV so I can laugh?" They joke about that when we get together all these years later. I even took a laughter yoga workshop recognizing I don't laugh enough. How about you?

CHAPTER 4

Thinking, Thinking, Thinking

"There is no illness of the body, apart from the mind."

-Socrates

"All that we are is the result of what we have thought. The mind is everything. What we think, we become."

-Buddha

"We are disturbed not by what happens to us but by our thoughts about what happens."

-Epictetus

When you were a child and kids made fun of you, as kids do, do you remember yelling, *"Sticks and stones will break my bones, but words will never hurt me?"* Were you bold enough to say the words? Or did you mumble, intimidated, "Sticks and stones...?" On some level, you knew that the words you were claiming did not hurt, in fact, did hurt—a lot. Words that hurt are not restricted to coming from the mouths of kids. The adults, knowingly or unknowingly, uttered hurtful words too. Can you hear them now? "Big girls don't cry." "Children should be seen and not heard." "Who do you think you are?" "Look at that B and C," as they missed all the A's, or they were too busy to look at the report and you—a little child looking for approval or simply to be seen. "I love you." "You are bad." Two messages, maybe heard daily. Which to believe? Then there are the other messages repeated over and over. My mom's mantra was, "Don't say anything because it might be the wrong thing." How do you learn to deal with life's inevitable conflicts with that tape playing?

Much later, I heard other hurtful words in the world of work. "Why are you taking a job from a man when you have a husband?" Some of you remember the cultural message many years ago for women about how to dress for success by dressing like a man? How many have heard this? "I do not love you anymore. I want a divorce." Maybe you are already feeling the memories of messages like these in your body— words from long ago that get stored in the cells like fat. Those words hurt, and we became angry. We armored up. We became numb. We pretended we were fine and buried our feelings. And pile on more of these kinds of cultural messages of society, of churches too. Do this, don't do that. Believe this, no, believe this, they are wrong. The words, the messages became pieces of our foundation. Words heard became how we see ourselves, how we think, the foundation of our thoughts and beliefs to this day, unless somehow, we have become awakened to who we really are. My mom also had another wonderful reminder, "If you can't say anything kind, don't say it." I now might add, "If you can't think anything kind, don't think it!"

Let's talk about perceptions. What are you seeing here in this classic trompe l'oeil? Two views? AND both right! Each of us perceives a situation, an event based upon perception. Mmmmm. A perfect moment for memories and insights at this point as we dive more deeply into the wellness journey.

Let's segue to the present. Thinking, thinking, thinking. More words, just not spoken! Where did the words come from? Did emotions precede them? Probably. The effect is the same. When you wake up in the morning, what are your first thoughts? A continuation of the stream from the day before, and the day before that? The current of thoughts, and the beliefs which develop from the thoughts we think over and over, have a powerful chemical effect on the body. Our negative thinking, which may stem from childhood messages heard over and over and over like those you just read, may be worse than germs with respect to stress and inflammation in the body. To the list of chronic diseases mentioned earlier, let's add the epidemic of self-criticism and criticism of others. We have to heal the mind, detox old emotions and traumas in order to be healthy and to thrive. Keep asking yourself, "Which thought feels better? Which thought feels better?"

Three years into my commitment to get healthy, I could answer, "How are you feeling?" with a 5 or 6 on the 10-point scale, certainly up from the 2 or 3. I was eating so much differently, but not as well as I am today, sleeping better, and my commitment to exercise never waned. I learned that the old cultural mindset that the "right" someone could fix me was false. I came to understand that substituting often very beneficial integrative healing practices such as acupuncture, homeopathy, chiropractic care, or taking fistfuls of supplements did not excuse me from doing the work of nourishing my body and mind. There had to be more steps I was not yet aware of to support my commitment to move higher on the scale, which works for me to this day to help me access how I am really feeling—a way of taking my pulse.

Another wakeup light flashed on when I was driving across Washington D.C.'s 14th Street Bridge early one gray winter morning on the way to my Baltimore office. I was thinking, thinking, thinking about my daughter. Truthfully, I was filled with fear given the path she was on. On top of that, I was thinking, thinking, thinking about all that I had to do at work, and about certain people who were not kind, to put it in my mom's terms. I was often insecure about all that was expected of me by others **and** myself! That, too, may be an epidemic, for I have heard other successful professional women utter similar feelings. And yes, I was still thinking about how to feel better. All these thoughts in only the first fifteen minutes of my drive! You can see why the mind is often referred to the monkey mind.

On this particular morning, I chose to turn the radio off when I reached the bridge, and it was as though my mind became tuned to a new station, an understanding from deep within! I instantly felt and knew that I had to change my thinking to achieve the level of wellbeing I knew was possible. How was that going to happen? I knew, intuitively now, that the answers and teachers would show up given my experiences of these past three years. And the bridge became a metaphor for me for crossing to this new stage of my life and healing from within.

My morning had started an hour earlier with a stream of really negative thinking and stressing that I, in these moments, realized had been my pattern for years, and the pattern of so many people I knew. Each morning, even before I opened my clenched eyes, the stream, actually more like a flood, of negative thinking started over again. The racing thoughts went like this: Too much to do, my daughter, my son, my boyfriend, how to fit in time to visit parents, grocery shop, and clean, work—the anxiety never stopped. Really, nearly the same thoughts, perhaps in different contexts, over and over, just as the data I later discovered told me was the repetitive pattern or nature of the mind… until it isn't!

I recalled how for years I called my best friend several mornings each week to just get going. Maybe there was the need to just connect with another loving adult with whom I felt safe. In my visit to memory lane, as I experienced a commute like never before, I saw in my mind the little gatherings in the halls of the office buildings over the years as people whispered judgments of colleagues and complained about who did what to whom in their lives. I have to acknowledge reluctantly that I participated in these gatherings at different stages of my career. Who knew that when you are pointing a finger at someone, there are three pointing back at yourself? Try that if you have not already. Who knew that those conversations were creating more stress?

There were other familiar patterns as I mulled over my insight during my hour drive. I recalled the weekly walk along the beautiful

Potomac with a friend to get our exercise. One of us told our story of "hard" life experiences of the week as we left the parking lot, and the other, her story of "hard" on the way back. You know the "hard"— your version of what I have already described. In the big picture, our lives were not "hard." It just felt that way at the time. For goodness sake, how many people in America get to walk along the Potomac with views of the Capitol, the Jefferson Memorial, and the planes not far over our heads as they landed at National Airport? We completely missed the peace, the calm, and the possibilities that were all around us. We could have laughed, been silly, or at least had some balance, but we did not know then. If we did not know, how could the walks have been different? Instead, we were in our familiar head space, and in our emotional pain bodies that Eckhart Tolle refers to. Yet, sometimes you have to get the pain out. By telling our story, there is often an understanding or insight that we might not have had otherwise, just as I am receiving additional understanding of my life experiences as I tell my story in this book. And I had not expected this. To tell your story or not is a paradox, because although it is important to acknowledge pain, it is just as important not to keep repeating stories of pain or we don't heal.

I knew without a doubt by the time I arrived in Baltimore that morning that I had to begin to tell a different story not only about my body, but about everything and everyone troubling me. Now, how to do it? How would I go about changing the thoughts and the stories I had been telling myself for a lifetime and that others had been telling me? I began to read self-help books, listen to CDs (actually, cassettes then). I turned off the news, at least while I was eating. Last year, I canceled cable news and the newspaper. Change continues as I become aware and am ready. Going more deeply, one morning, I woke up and decided to practice non-judgment for the day. That means non-judgment of anyone, including myself. Try this experiment and see how long you can go. Look in the mirror when you wake up and don't judge. That is a good start. You might even tell yourself, "I love myself so much." It will feel awkward, silly even, until you realize how good it feels—as though your body, heart, and mind have been craving those words for so long. Release any thought that focusing on you is selfish!

What we feed our bodies with our thoughts or mumbled words is critical to health. Remember the lifetime of feelings, thoughts, or memories long buried—the ones that tell you you're not good enough, or the ones that say I "gotta" be more, do more. I recall my unconscious habit of walking rather fast down the long halls of my office building under the illusion I could accomplish more with speed. Then, there was the moment when a young woman who emptied my office trash each day with a smile, no less, helped me to empty some trash in my thinking. She gently asked, "Why do you always walk so fast with your head down?" UHH, I had no idea! In that moment, she was my teacher, offering a wakeup that I could hear, probably after so many that I could not hear. Such a gift. I slowed a bit, and I have consciously practiced looking forward, not down, ever since.

Years later, I was in southeastern France in one of the few large stores, almost like our Target. I observed a man, perhaps an immigrant from northern Africa, on his hands and knees scrubbing the floor of a public bathroom. He was singing, yes, singing, as he did the work he probably did every day—work that many of us would complain about. Perhaps he was simply grateful to be in France, grateful to have a job. And again, I thanked the lady who reminded me about the way I went about my day so many years before. It is all a choice.

Another teacher taught me that when we give eighteen seconds of airtime to the negative, we are feeding more thinking in the same vein. It becomes hard to get out of that cycle. I began to really understand the potential damage of words, thoughts, and beliefs when I heard about highly successful people who were eating right, sleeping, exercising, but still experiencing life threatening illnesses. I realized that how I nourished my body with my thoughts, beliefs, and emotions is an integral piece of the healing puzzle.

Practice. Then. Practice Some More to Change the Story and to Lighten Your Load.

Accept that we are born to experience a complex array of emotions. How could we appreciate love without its absence? Peace without having experienced stress? Laughter and joy without tears? We live in a society where it is uncomfortable, even unacceptable to confront grief, fear, and anxiety. About forty years ago, Senator Edmund Muskie, a highly respected Senator from Maine, my childhood state, was running for the Democratic Party's nomination for president. He became teary when a media outlet criticized his wife. Those tears were a major factor in abruptly ending his campaign as nearly the entire national media jumped in to portray his show of emotion as evidence of instability. Do you think that tearing up would be acceptable today? Are emotions acceptable?

What about guilt? Have you ever been accused of just trying to make someone feel guilty with tears? Emotions are real. Sometimes there is even guilt around fun and play. For years, I cringed when someone said, "Have fun." What was the memory or experience that produced that belief? When my mom was in her nineties and experiencing dementia, she slowly got out the words, "Have fun while you can, dear." Perhaps she was seeing her daughter being too serious, working too hard. Maybe she was remembering her life, and from her photos as a young woman, it looked as though she had a lot of fun. I was a product of northern New England where the ethos was hard work before pleasure. MMMM. What about you? What were you taught?

Grief we cannot deny, cannot bury. FEEL the FEELINGS. Don't stuff them. When you are grieving and you feel like the sky is falling and your body cannot stop trembling, cry until there are no more tears. Then, cry some more, ignoring the voice in your head telling you not to cry because you are "big." Maybe scream too. You cannot skip over powerful emotions. After a while, perhaps a long while, the tears will dry up. And then the feelings will surface again and again with less intensity each time as we heal. Try to find some good in each day during these times. Invite and allow lots of support from family, friends, and counselors. You cannot go from being at the lowest level of the emotional ladder to joy in these circumstances, but you can go from grief to appreciation. Whatever you do, don't go it alone to show how strong you are.

Catch yourself repeating the same old victim stories. Consider seeking help to fully feel your feelings. I have found the Emotional Freedom Technique (EFT) and more recently, Thought Field Therapy (TFT) extremely powerful. I experienced some discomfort or pain in a shoulder for three years. Yoga, physical therapy, and wishing it or visualizing it away had not worked completely. TFT practiced for one hour was literally a miracle during a ride from Tulum, Mexico to Cancun. Occasionally, if I feel a twinge, a couple minutes of TFT is all that is necessary! Working with a highly trained practitioner helps to free grief or trauma and pain or judgment from the cells where old memories that block the flow of energy are stored. You can also learn online, but I found that I was not motivated to do the "work" by myself... until I was. You will be surprised how one conscious memory gives rise to so many more unconscious memories that need to be released for the health of your body. Words, thoughts, and memories are all energy. Everything is energy. Did you know that? Just as a stream blocked by the handiwork of a hardworking beaver family cannot flow, our own energy cannot flow and support our life force if it is blocked by old memories, physical injuries, and the damage being done by highly processed food-junk. See how it all ties together?

Set one day for observation. Where does you mind wander naturally? To optimism or fear, stress, judgment, or humor and creativity? Notice what you like about people, not what you don't. Observe where your mind goes to feed itself. Do you like what you observe? These changes take practice, so be gentle on yourself.

Remember when I suggested cleaning out the kitchen and bathroom cabinets? Well, now you get to clear out the thought clutter cabinet. You can have only one thought in each moment. What will be your focus? How will you nourish yourself with your thoughts?

All Those Stressors and Physical Effects

If you are experiencing physical manifestations from the stressors such as frequent colds, depression, insomnia, or any chronic disease, even the shoulder pain I mentioned, begin to notice your thought patterns. If anyone asks you, "Where does stress start?" it seems the answer is in the head. True, but only in part. Hormones change, the heart beats faster, cortisol affects the blood vessels, and your brain connects with your gut (your second brain), and leads to gut disease and more. Your whole immune system is under attack and epigenetic changes are occurring. Remember that lifestyle trumps genes according to the science of epigenetics. Remember, too, that stress causes the heightened inflammatory response noted in nearly all chronic disease. Of course, stress may be beneficial in situations of danger when we have to act or react. However, chronic stress is making us ill. Remember that stress from our thoughts and beliefs, our foods, and the toxins around us is the cause behind most chronic disease. Stress is a factor in weight and obesity. You can't dismiss this stress "thing" or the interconnectedness of getting moving, what you eat, sleep, your thoughts and beliefs to being healthy.

Ready for More Ideas for Reducing Stressors?

First, ask yourself if it is time, if you are ready to explore the possibilities of looking inward. Is this a missing link for you as it was for me? Or, ask if you are too busy to focus on this thinking and feeling stuff. Are you judging the whole concept? There is the "perception" idea again. Are you too distracted to even notice that your body is sending you signals every moment? Emotional and physical pain can be numbed with pills or food and busyness, but not for a lifetime. Even by referring to "my bad back," "my Crohn's," or "my arthritis," you are reinforcing the condition as yours. You are telling your body and mind that this condition belongs to you. Find different language such as "the pain in the back" or, "this diagnosis of cancer, not my cancer." Now, you are acknowledging it exists but not owning it. It has been mentioned earlier that when we acknowledge pain, we create an avenue for its release. Again, we are not denying what is in the moment.

- Ask if there are people in your life whom you are judging all the time, including yourself. Byron Katie, in *Loving What Is*, asks us to consider these four questions: "Is the thought or belief true? Can you absolutely know it is true? How do you react; what happens when you believe that thought? Who would you be without the thought?"[10]

- What if we look back at whatever is troubling you from the other's perspective? Maybe the person you are challenged by reminds you unconsciously of someone who was hard on you years ago? What if you looked for what someone does right instead of what you perceive as wrong, as you have read before? Maybe the real toxins are only, in part, the processed foods we eat, but the toxins that build a wall around our hearts when we judge and cannot speak our feelings with each other. Remember perceptions. Maybe you saw the faces of two women in the trompe l'oeil above and a friend saw the vase or glass—both of you are right! Is it possible that being able to see things from someone else's perspective may totally change your life?

- How about another story moment? Late last summer, my beautiful crepe myrtle, whose blossoms amazingly match the décor of my living room, began to naturally drop its flowers and let go. Each morning, I went out to sweep before the flowers could stain the steps of my circular stairs and deck. One morning, I have to admit, I was whining just a bit about having one more thing I had to do. Typically, just when I needed another teacher, she appeared. My neighbor in the townhouse next to mine came outside, and gazing at the blossoms that had fallen on her side of the fence on her steps, remarked, "It looks as though the angels were throwing a confetti party last night." Two perceptions—I chose hers with an inner smile and with much appreciation.

- Take a walk. Go to the movies. Watch your favorite sitcom. (Mine is The Big Bang Theory.) Find a friend to laugh with until you cry, or cry with this friend to release sadness. Play with some kids. Stay away from the complainers. Take a nap. Or, look again at what you are eating. Get a pet. We never judge our furry friends who leave lovely footprints on our hearts. Get an adult coloring book. Remember those connect the dot books to create a picture when we were kids? What we are doing here is connecting the dots, the pieces of the puzzle to create health… for life. Get a massage. Write for ten or twenty minutes daily, for several consecutive days, about any emotion. Finally, go to a Cancun beach!

With all of the focus on negative stress, did you know that not all stress is bad for you? Have you ever heard of eustress, which comes from the Greek prefix "eu" for healthy? Stress that comes from being able to accomplish something that you never thought you could, such as writing a first book, or lifting five pounds more than the week before represents a positive response to a stressor. Doing something that stresses you just a little helps you to grow so that things that used to stress you no longer do. Make sense? Hope and a sense of meaning and wellbeing accompany eustress. Thinking about all the pieces of the healing puzzle can seem daunting, stressful in a negative way. Yet, you start in, and the result may be eustress as you see little results as you work with interconnected pieces of the healing puzzle: Exercise, sleep, foods, thoughts, a whole new way of nourishing yourself. One more piece of the puzzle is coming after these contemplations.

Two Contemplations

- Dr. Viktor Frankl, Holocaust survivor and author of *Man's Search for Meaning,* wrote, "Everything can be taken away from a man but one thing: The last of the human freedoms—to choose one's attitude in any given set of circumstances, to choose one's own way."

- Two Wolves. A Native American grandfather is talking to his grandson about how he feels about a tragedy in the village. The grandfather is saying, "I feel as if I have two wolves fighting in my heart. One wolf is the vengeful, angry, violent one. The other wolf is the loving, compassionate one." The little boy asks, "Grandfather, which wolf will win the fight in your heart?" The grandfather places his hand on his heart and replies, "The one I feed."

CHAPTER 5

"It Is Safe to Open Your Heart, You Know"

"We only need to take the first step beyond all that we have known for reality to begin to unfold itself before us. We need to take that first step not once, but continually evermore."

-Adyashanti

"And now here is my secret, a very simple secret. It is only with the heart one can see rightly; what is essential is invisible to the eye."

-Antoine de Saint-Exupery

D uring what came to be my last year in the Federal Service, I had never been so inspired or become so disappointed. I placed my knowledge and the deep caring in my heart into a proposal based upon another reoccurring insight that the integrative health practices I had been studying could benefit a large population of disability recipients and save millions of dollars which Americans were paying into Social Security trust funds too. I submitted a proposed feasibility project following a series of meetings with leading medical experts over the year. When politics precluded the feasibility study from happening, I chose to "retire" early and return to sunny southern California. I left the East Coast with two clear intentions: To help make a difference in the health of people from that end of the country, and of course, to live happily ever after. Once again, my life went in a direction I could never have predicted or imagined. So much for those five year plans I labored over so long ago from *What Color Is Your Parachute?*

I prepared deliberately, and yes, I admit, feverishly, at the same time, for leaving the East Coast once again—this time in a more permanent way than I had in my planned one-year escape and exploration in the late 1980s. This time, I sold my house, my car, and lots of furniture. To relax a bit as I was bringing together all the pieces of this latest transition, I decided on a beach weekend and a yoga class in nearby Delaware. This yoga class was unlike any yoga class I had taken since I began to add yoga to my life only a few months earlier in the hopes of helping with lingering aches, pains, and stresses.

When I started going to the weekly classes at my gym, the practice was so foreign to our culture that people who went to yoga were considered strange. Accordingly, because I did not want to be judged for being different, or any more different than I was already being considered with my new ideas, I told no one where I was going. Stealth yoga, eh! At the gym I practiced a variety of yoga styles that included lots of action and rigidly held poses. Rigid was exactly what I did not need, but I did not know that then. The beach yoga was certainly the opposite style. I "rested" on blankets in easy poses most of the ninety-minute class while my mind was repeating, "Waste of time, not doing anything." When I stood up, however, I was astounded. I realized I had never felt this experience of openness, even stillness and ease, ever. I almost wondered if I still had a body. I felt that light. As a reminder of life's synchronicities and "when the student is ready" concept, I also discovered that day that yoga teacher training for this yoga style was offered in La Jolla, not far from my ultimate destination of Los Angles. Right then and there, I decided to take the one-month, fourteen-hour-a-day training before I moved to Los Angeles. At the same time, I clearly believed that I had no intention of teaching. So it was without any hesitation that on the first day of training, I replied in response to why I was there with, "Well, it is for me." I even recall the guilt of acknowledging that awareness when nearly everyone was sharing their mission to teach and to serve others. Well, I have been teaching now for sixteen years! Never say, "Never." Clichés and truisms exist for a reason. I also came to understand that I had to heal myself on a deeper level before I could serve others.

Yoga and Meditation

Yoga has been being practiced for thousands of years in India. Any practice that has been embraced for so long and finally here in this country where twenty-one million adults and nearly two million children attend classes must be powerful. Whether we practice for health, fitness, how we look, or for spiritual awakening, you will get what you need at the time from the commitment to practice. I admit I fit into the first three of these categories when I arrived in La Jolla. Only a minority of people in this country would say yoga is about discovering who you are deep inside. For me, that awareness began to come gradually with the cumulative effects of the physical and emotional changes from training and years of practice combined with all the reading I was doing from the books of Wayne Dyer, Deepak Chopra, Marianne Williamson, and so many more, along with the yogic spiritual texts. If you decide you are ready to add yoga to your life, I recommend finding a teacher and a practice that works for you at this stage in your life. Please be careful in your choices that you do not cause yourself injury. I can assure you that a gentle restorative yoga might be best no matter your age. Hint: Could there be strength in learning to let go?

During the first few days of training, I began to discover how tight my body really was. Also, we were meditating—an integral aspect of yoga. I had never gone back to meditating after the morning wakeup call on the Cancun beach seven years before. I was so busy focusing on exercising and learning some of what you have been reading about in this little book that I had never really given much thought to going within. Moreover, I really did not understand then what that meant. Because I was physically uncomfortable sitting on a stack of blankets in the middle of the yoga room, attempting the meditation that some of the students seemed so comfortable with, I joined a few others in the back of the room to use the wall for support, as the teacher suggested. On the second or third day, when it seemed I could not sit still another moment, I heard, *"It is safe to open your heart, you know."* Oh, oh, once again, words that were not my words. And as with the Cancun wakeup, here I was, being given guidance I was unable to ignore and did not want to ignore. I felt these words represented the next message for my healing as an inner journey. I experienced these words so gently in contrast to the words on the beach. Those in Cancun felt more like an alarm. These were like saying, "Honey, you can soften that armor you think protects you from the pain." That armor was preventing me from really living and experiencing all the emotions we are here to experience.

The meaning of this message did not allude me. The familiar poses done so differently in the Svaroopa style were already reaching into those frozen places in my body, frozen from falls and other accidents, the *"sticks and stones."* Stuck energy gets trapped around our organs and leads to disease. Did you know that? There began to be moments in the day when tears flowed until I thought they would not stop. I was not alone. Nearly all the teacher trainees experienced profound releases. Our teacher explained that we did not have to know the reason why the ice was melting, but to just allow the body to open, the emotions to flow. Our hearts were opening!

In our culture, doctors may recommend these practices to lower blood pressure or to feel better. In the east, meditation was prescribed for enlightenment. Even if results seem initially invisible to you, Dr. Deepak Chopra says meditation helps us to make better decisions, to deal with stress, to less likely be discouraged, and to become more creative and optimistic. Moreover, the study of epigenetics is revealing how meditation supports the body and the mind, even slowing the aging process. Start by sitting for ten minutes at lunch-time with your eyes closed, or take a few conscious breaths several times daily. Then, increase your meditation time and teach your children. Tip: Stop your car a block or so from home to get in fifteen minutes of meditation. At some point, you may want to go to a meditation retreat.

So many books, DVDs, and online programs are available to teach you different versions of the best ways to meditate. My advice is not to take time initially to study recommendations about the perfect meditation technique. Instead, just jump in! Commit to a daily time to just sit or walk quietly until you naturally and regularly start to notice your breath and your body, and to allow the moment to be just as it is. Dr. Chopra says that if you think you don't have time to meditate once a day, you should meditate twice a day! While thoughts almost never stop completely for long because the nature of the mind is to think, you begin to revel in each moment of sitting and listening and living your life. The benefits of yoga and meditation really do become cumulative. And you begin to find moments in your life where there is no separation between prayer time, meditation time, and the work you are doing. Really!

The opening of my heart and body has continued for sixteen years, taking me further into the mystery of life–what is hidden in each of our hearts. Ancient societies and cultures understood more about the human heart than we who have thought of it almost exclusively as a physical pump. The ancients understood the heart to be the seat of the soul, the source of a deep love beyond the sentimentality we often ascribe to the heart. Science is now increasingly confirming what these spiritual traditions have been teaching us—that our heart's deeper intelligence is real and is important to our health and our sense of meaning. Through the commitment to yoga and meditation, we support the release of trapped emotions affecting our wellbeing, discussed in the *Thinking, Thinking, Thinking* chapter–emotions that create a wall around the heart. I began to understand that the physical healing road and the spiritual healing road are parallel roads taken together. The paths merge along the way to become one.

Qigong

Shortly after I completed yoga teacher training, I was introduced to Qigong in southern California. In my way of being open to new ideas and practices, or living a bit beyond my comfort zone, I decided to take a weekend training. While the weekend was extraordinary, I instinctively felt I could not embrace yoga and Qigong, two new practices simultaneously. For thirteen years, I never thought of Qigong again. Then, Qigong and the teacher Mingtong Gu kept crossing my mind. As I now understand, when memory flashes reoccur, I am being asked to pay attention. I was not surprised to find myself on a plane headed to San Francisco last spring, having once again responded to the nudges and pulls for another one-month training, this time in Wisdom Healing Qigong.

Let me tell you that these kinds of experiences bring up every resistance stored in the body, mind, and heart. There were many times in both trainings I wanted to leave, to escape, but knew I could not. Each night I rolled into my bed after another day of fourteen hours of Qigong training wanting to call the airlines to book a flight home the next day. Everything was new, and yet there was such an obvious relationship to the yoga I had faithfully practiced for years. My emotions were raw as areas in my body where energy was blocked began to release, just as in the yoga training fifteen years before. At the Qigong retreat, which was so different from the yoga training where the students were physically healthy, I watched people with severe Parkinson's experience small improvements within two weeks. One man went from needing his wife to feed him to managing a spoon himself. Another woman in her fifties, participating in her third or fourth retreat with Mingtong, told me she had had advanced Parkinson's that required her to leave her executive job. Now, the only remaining evidence of the disease was slight trembling in her left arm. Of course, she practiced several hours a day to restore her to wellness.

I was humbled by the courage of so many of the participants. I stayed, of course. Nine months later, I continue to practice daily. I am happier than ever. My heart is more open and I wear a deeper inner smile that accompanies my outer smile that for so many years of my life was a mask for how I was really feeling. I also frequently remind myself to lift my heart. Notice what you feel when you lift your heart. Was Qigong what I needed to release additional layers of very old, unconscious "stuff?" Did this opening and letting go experience allow me to begin to give birth to this book that has been in me for several years? Timing and readiness can be so difficult to understand, as life itself. Qigong and yoga will be as much a part of my life as healthy eating or any other self-care, nourishing practices for the rest of my life.

The quotes from the *Healing Process* by Master Mingtong Gu express so profoundly what Qigong offers. "Qigong invites us to experience our life story through the writings it has left on our muscles, nerves, organs, emotions, and energy flow. The powerful Qigong tool of sound helps restore and cultivate harmony within an organ system at the cellular level. When we activate the vibration for the liver through sound, for example, we transform the old programming of anger to a new feeling of courage and clarity of mind. Our historic response (genetic and attitude) now has a new choice of cultivating harmony so that we can move through the world of family, friends, work and home in a more positive and happy way and healthy way."

It's All Energy

Are you beginning to understand that your body is energy? Are you beginning to understand, if you did not already, what you are really saying when you exclaim, "I have no energy!" Everything is energy. Nikola Tesla said, "If you want to know the secrets of the universe, think in terms of energy, frequency and vibration." I don't have a favorite book to recommend that you curl up with that tells you all about quantum physics and your body being energy. Instead, I recommend you experiment with energy for yourself by bringing your elbows to your sides and your lower arms parallel to the earth. Ever so slowly, bring your hands a bit closer, then back, and repeat until you feel a tingling, vibration, or heat. That is energy. The first time you experience this field, you know you have traveled a long way from the powerlessness of, "I have no energy."

Recently, I shared this experiment with my grandsons. Sean, the almost eight-year-old, with wide eyes of surprise, grinned at me and exclaimed, "N'annie, I feel it." A couple moments later he added, "I have more energy."

Energy is limitless. Leap to knowing what you can do for your own body, a field of energy capable of shifting its vibrations through every thought, every food, all that you do. Through my practice of yoga and Qigong, I began to tap into this subtle energy. Once you touch this field, you will never feel the same. Just as we are proving all this with "modern" science, the yogis, the Qigong masters, the Christian mystics knew this all along.

Intellectually, I understand there are layers inside the body beyond the physical. Let's go back to the heart, which is the first organ to form, not the brain. The heart's electrical field is about sixty times stronger than the currents of the brain. The electromagnetic field of your heart extends about three feet beyond your body. And "electromagnetic signals generated by the heart have the capacity to affect others around us"[11]. You may even begin to understand why we have expressions like halfhearted, openhearted, heart to heart, and brokenhearted. It is safe and necessary to open your heart to allow energy to flow without blockages in order to enjoy the health you are meant to enjoy. And it is necessary to allow the flow of energy through every organ in our bodies by nourishing ourselves through movement, healthy food choices, enough sleep, and positive thoughts and beliefs. Then, there is the essential, deeper self-care from within—a newer concept in our culture, but such an ancient concept in eastern cultures, that nourishes us and heals us. Meditation, yoga, and Qigong are keys to allowing the flow of healing energy and allowing the heart to be wide open.

"The Foundation Is Laid"

"We are guests at Life's table, where the food is of our choosing."

-Alice Fancher

"Two roads diverged in a yellow wood, and I, I took the one less traveled by and that has made all the difference."

-Robert Frost

I n the days following my life changing month of yoga teacher training, I anticipated my new beginnings from my light-filled apartment, looking out over the distant blue water of Marina del Rey. What I did not anticipate was the construction of a high-rise in the field filled with colorful wild flowers that was my close-up view, along with the sea a little further—the view that had sealed the deal for me to move in the month before. This was the serene scene I had dreamed of during the ten years I lived back east. Instead, the dirt, the noise, and fumes of idling trucks and earth diggers from early morning to dusk caused me to play victim. Who does not know the, "Why is this happening to me?" refrain. And over the months, I self-diagnosed that I was in a dark night of the soul, not just because of the construction, however. I journaled, I cried, I reached out to old friends, I got a bit of counseling, I ate chocolate doughnuts, I walked the beach, and I was so hard on myself for not appreciating my life.

When I started the letting go process years before with my commitment to heal, I had no idea what to expect, but this was not it! I didn't even have the vocabulary that included, "letting go!" Life in California was causing me to explore more deeply. Nearly two years into this darkness, amidst the sunshine on the outside, I realized one morning as I walked the beach that the building of the high-rise, from its beginning to the steel beams just being raised, was a metaphor for my life. I had to leave everyone and everything on the East Coast to experience an emptiness I could never have experienced had I stayed. I had to dig out the dirt, or at least allow the dirt to surface, and to lay the foundation for the rest of my life. One evening, about three years after moving to California, the words, *"The foundation is laid,"* came to me during the deep relaxation of shavasana, the last fifteen minutes of yoga class. I had to keep repeating those words all the way up the hill to my apartment in La Jolla, where I was now living. I knew this was another message with a significant meaning. My third message, and I so grateful. Not until I reached the top of the hill was I able to connect the words with my partial understanding of why I was in California that I had experienced on the beach walk a year before. I was there to build a new foundation and had been "told" that the foundation was laid. I burst into deep sobs of gratitude. Since it was already 9pm and three hours later on the East Coast, I had to wait until the next morning to call my daughter to say, "Your mom is coming home, honey."

The Pieces of the Puzzle

*"Remember, the entrance door to the
sanctuary is inside you."*

-Rumi

*"We live our lives forward and understand
them backward."*

-Kierkegaard

*"Your own self-realization is the greatest gift
you can give this world."*

-Maharishi

The journey of *Looking for Health in All the Right Places* has brought us to an eye-opening, heart-opening discovery of possibilities for a new vision, a greater vision of life as we each choose consciously how to put the pieces of our life's puzzle together. Our old programming is set free. This journey becomes one of knowing ultimately, I feel, that we are in the "right places" when we realize that life is an inside journey of self-love, and health is the gift of this path. The old way of looking outside fades away as we lay the new foundation. The open heart is the way. An open heart breeds courage, patience, and self-love. Though it takes practice, when we keep an open heart, we can embrace our deepest feelings and nurture our true selves.

What I have discovered is that the first step is to acknowledge that it is time for a change, then the looking and seeking, then the finding and knowing. The journey, which may take a moment or years, is followed by a period of what I call "integration of the shifts," the changes and a sense of, "Oh, I have got it." Then more looking and finding. This is life. The searching, the finding, then more. I discovered along the way that the internal changes even came to be reflected in how I saw myself and how others saw me when I was Anna, then Ann, and after California, Annie. Who could guess, even imagine all of this.

You are holding pieces of my story that may influence you, stir you to focus on your story, your own puzzle pieces, the story and the wakeup call your body has been telling you, as mine had. And you are holding what I know from these twenty-three years of study and practice is how to create a healthy and happier you. You have so many of the pieces for nourishing yourself, for feeding yourself with exercise, unprocessed foods, sleep, your thoughts and beliefs, for opening your heart with meditation, yoga or Qigong. I cannot write a recipe or a prescription for you of what to do first or second, nor can I tell you to jump in and do as much as you can as soon as you can. However, if you ask yourself what is yours to do in this moment, if you are open and ready, you will get a sensation, a feeling in your gut, in your heart, somewhere in your body when you begin to ask and say that you are ready for the next step. Or there may be a nudge that you can't identify, or a symptom that won't go away that is telling you that there must be a shift.

Just be aware that there is no secret to health and longevity in seven easy steps or just ten or twenty things to do for happiness and health. Please also understand that being human does not mean being completely consistent all the time, and life may mean going in many directions all at the same time. I have paused often and both embraced and resisted the contradictions of my humanity, as you have read in these pages. Are there lessons to learn? Oh, yes. Choose to bring together the voices you hear from the outside and inside. Question and invite in what resonates for you now, a weaving of the tapestry or the story you are writing.

Culturally, we are accustomed to looking for the shortcut and for someone to tell us what to do. You are the author of your life. What will you choose today? What is the story you are going to write knowing that how you are living today is, in fact, writing your healthy story, or not? There may be an insight, one moment that will lead you in a new direction, the road you could never have imagined the day before, the road that makes all the difference in laying the foundation for your next chapter, and the next. And a few years or months or days from now, there will be another nudge, another shift, and another floor added to your solid foundation. You are holding your life in your hands. Your life is precious. Your body is precious. I predict there are a few pieces of the puzzle that will remain a mystery until you have lived the lessons.

I heard Maurice Sendak, author of the book, *Where the Wild Things Are,* a book you may have read as a child or read to your kids, offer these words of wisdom a few months before his death at eighty-three: *"Live your life; live your life; live your life.* What an opportunity for a grand design and transformation many times over. Taste the possibilities. Feel the possibilities!

I will not die an unlived life.
I will not live in fear
Of falling or catching fire.
I choose to inhabit my days,
To allow my living to open me,
To make me less afraid,
More accessible,
To loosen my heart
Until it becomes a wing,
A torch, a promise.
I choose to risk my significance;
To live
So that which came to me as seed
Goes to the next as blossom
And that which came
To me as blossom,
Goes on as fruit.

-Dawna Markova

Your Story—Now, Your Turn

*"A year from now what will you wish
you had done today?"*

-Liam Linisong

*"Just when the caterpillar thought the world was over,
it became a butterfly."*

-Proverb

*"It's your road, and yours alone; others may walk it with
you; but no one can walk it for you."*

- Rumi

A Few Questions for You to Consider

How am I feeling today? _____

_____

_____

Why do I want to feel differently?_____

_____

_____

What am I ready to do differently?_____

_____

_____

What number do I intend to be on the 10-point scale and by when?

Number:_____

Date: _____

How committed am I to myself?_____

_____

_____

Create Your Own Journal

Puzzle Pieces for Each Day:

How I am nourishing myself with movement? _____

_____

_____

How I am nourishing myself with my food choices? _____

_____

_____

How I am nourishing myself with sleep? _____

_____

_____

How I am nourishing myself with my thoughts and beliefs? _____

_____

_____

How am I nourishing myself with deeper self-care: Meditation, yoga, or Qigong? _____

_____

_____

What am I grateful for in this moment? _____

_____

_____

What am I noticing and feeling as I go along? _____

_____

_____

Choices I made that did not serve me: _____

_____

_____

Every 30 Days
(At least until the new ways are established and integrated.)

Where am I? What am I noticing from the pieces of the puzzle I have been focusing on? Am I acknowledging my progress? _____

_____

_____

_____

_____

Where do I need to be? _____

_____

_____

_____

_____

Do I need an accountability partner, a physical check-up, an integrative health counselor, a yoga or Qigong teacher, EFT practitioner? OR? _____

_____

WRITING your accomplishments and your intentions is your own contract with yourself.

You Might Want to Explore Further

Books I Cherish*

Super Genes
Deepak Chopra, MD, and Rudolph Tanzi, PhD

Wheat Belly, Total Health
William Davis, MD

Women, Food, and God
Geneen Roth

Hidden Messages in Water
Masaru Emoto

Broken Open
Elizabeth Lesser

Loving What Is
Byron Katie

Biology of Belief
Bruce Lipton

Falling Into Grace
Adyashanti (Choose any of his books.)

A New Way to Be Human
Robert Taylor

Power of Now or A New Earth
Eckhart Tolle

Hero's Journey
Joseph Campbell

The Alchemist
Paulo Coelho

* So many new books are in print. These are my favorites. You will find your own favorites too for this inside journey.

Web Sources

www.mercola.com

www.thetruthaboutcancer.com

www.greenmedinfo.com

www.ewg.org

www.cornucopia.org

www.chicenter.com

www.mommypotamus.com (Check site for information on reducing EMF exposure)

www.wiredchild.org

www.draxe.com

www.healthychild.org

www.heartmath.org

Film

Inside Out

Cookware

Xtrema

Le Crueset

Works Cited

[1]"Nearly 7 in 10 Americans Take Prescription Drugs, Mayo Clinic, Olmsted Medical Center Find." *Mayonewsreleases.* Mayo Clinic, 19 June 2013. Web.

[2]Kliff, Sarah. "The U.S. Ranks 26th for Life Expectancy, Right Behind Slovenia." Washington Post. WP Company, LLC, 21 November 2013. Web.

[3]Kane, Jason. "Health Costs: How the U.S. Compares With Other Countries." PBS Newshour. WQED, 22 October 2012. Web.

[4]Environmental Working Group. "Body Burden: The Pollution in Newborns." *EWG.* EWG, 14 July 2005. Web.

[5]Geggel, Laura. "Too Much Sitting Is Killing You (Even If You Exercise)." *HumanOrigins.* Livescience, 21 January 2015. Web.

[6]Goldschmidt, Vivian. "Debunking The Milk Myth: Why Milk Is Bad For You And Your Bones." *Save Our Bones.* Save Institute, n.d. Web.

[7]Ghose, Tia. "Low-Fiber Diet May Change Gut Microbes for Generations." *Human Origins.* Livescience, 19 January 2016. Web.

[8]U.S. EPA. "Air and Radiation: Basic Information." *United States Environmental Protection Agency.* U.S. EPA, 23 February 2016. Web.

[9]WHO. "Electromagnetic Fields and Public Health: Mobile Phones." *World Health Organization. WHO,* October 2014. Web.

[10]Katie, Byron. *Loving What Is.* New York City: Three Rivers Press, 2003. Print.

[11]HeartMath Institute. "The Energetic Heart Is Unfolding." *Science of the Heart. HeartMath* Institute, 22 July 2010. Web.